ABBREVIATIONS IN MEDICINE

Abbreviations in Medicine

FOURTH EDITION

Edwin B. Steen, Ph.D.

*Professor Emeritus of Anatomy and Physiology
Western Michigan University*

BAILLIÈRE TINDALL · LONDON

A BAILLIÈRE TINDALL book published by
Cassell & Co Ltd
35 Red Lion Square, London WC1R 4SG
and at Sydney, Auckland, Toronto, Johannesburg
an affiliate of
Macmillan Publishing Co. Inc.
New York

First published 1960
Third edition 1971
Fourth edition 1978

ISBN 0 7020 0667 X

Phototypeset in VIP Helvetica by
Western Printing Services Ltd, Bristol

Printed in Great Britain by
Billing & Sons Ltd, Guildford, London and Worcester

CONTENTS

PREFACE

It was apparent several years ago that the widespread use of abbreviations in medical literature had reached a point where a handy source of reference had become a necessity. The original edition of this dictionary, the first of its kind in the field of medicine and the related sciences, was published in the United States in 1960 in the hope that it would fulfil that need and, at the same time, help to introduce a measure of standardization into an otherwise chaotic field. The success of that edition, and of its successors, has now led to the need for a fourth edition.

The scope of the dictionary has been extensively widened by adding new abbreviations from nearly every field of medicine. These include additional abbreviations of medical organizations, terms used in dentistry, occupational and physical therapy, cardiorespiratory therapy, and other specialized fields. Abbreviations of many new biochemical terms now used in medicine have been added. Especial attention has been given to the inclusion of new abbreviations employed in various laboratory procedures and reports and in the everyday operation of hospitals and clinics.

Because of the large number of new abbreviations encountered in the preparation of this revision, a degree of selection had to be employed as not all could be included. Abbreviations for short words, except for weights and measures, have been omitted as well as abbreviations for trite or trivial terms. Multiple abbreviations for the same term have been reduced in number. Some abbreviations for highly specialized terms having a restricted use are not listed. Abbreviations for terms identifying structures in illustrations appearing in texts or scientific papers are generally omitted.

Full stops separating the letters have been omitted from entries in line with the current trend of writing abbreviations without stops, and to avoid duplication (and pontification) where both styles are employed. Abbreviations are given throughout the book in capitals except where common usage dictates the use of small letters. Where there is more than one way of abbreviating a term, no attempt has been made to state which is correct, but simply to list all forms likely to be encountered. Needless to say, where there is any possibility of confusion in the context, words should be spelled out in full. The use of italic has been reserved for Latin terms defined in the dictionary and for scientific names of organisms.

I should like to thank those who have aided in the revision by calling attention to errors and suggesting new abbreviations to be listed. Especially appreciated were the contributions of Dr Adam G. N. Moore of Boston, Mass. and Dr R.J. Hetherington, of Birmingham, England. I am grateful also to the Upjohn Company, Bronson Methodist Hospital, the Borgess Hospital, and Western Michigan University, all of Kalamazoo, Michigan, and to the editorial staff of my publishers for their contributions and helpful suggestions.

September 1977   EDWIN B. STEEN

A

A:
absorbance (symbol for in spectrophotometry)
acceptor
acetum
adenine
adenosine
adrenaline
adult
allergy(ist)
alveolar gas
amphetamine
anaesthetic
anaphylaxis
Ångstrom unit
annum (L) year
anterior
aqueous
area (of heart shadow)
argon (chemical symbol for)
arteria

a:
accommodation
acid
acidity, total
ampere
anode
anterior
aqua (L) water
area
artery
asymmetric
atto (10^{-18})
axial

a:
alpha (first letter of Greek alphabet)
Symbol designating *first*
In organic compounds, refers to the carbon atom which is next to the carbon atom bearing the active group of molecules
Å: Ångstrom unit
A$_2$: aortic second sound
AA:
achievement age
Alcoholics Anonymous
amino acid
anticipatory avoidance
Associations of Anaesthetists
$\overline{\text{aa}}$, $\overline{\text{aa}}$: *ana* (Gr) of each
AAA:
abdominal aortic aneurysm
acute anxiety attack
American Academy of Allergy
American Academy of Anatomists
aaa: amalgam
AAALAC: American Association for Accreditation of Laboratory Animal Care
AAAS: American Association for the Advancement of Science
AABB: American Association of Blood Banks
AACHP: American Association for Comprehensive Health Planning
AACP: American Academy of Cerebral Palsy
AAD: alloxazine adenine dinucleotide (FAD)
AADP: American Academy of Dental Prosthetics
AADR: American Academy of Dental Radiology
AADS: American Academy of Dental Schools
AAE:
active assistive exercise
acute allergic encephalitis
American Association of Endodontists
AAF:
acetic-alcohol-formalin (a fixing fluid)
acetylaminofluorine
Army Air Force
ascorbic acid factor
AAFD: American Academy of Family Physicians
AAGP: American Academy of General Practice
AAHPER: American Academy for Health, Physical Education and Recreation
AAI: American Association of Immunologists
AAID: American Association of Implant Dentures

AAIN: American Association of Industrial Nurses

AAL: anterior axillary line

AALAS: American Association of Laboratory Animal Science

AAMA: American Academy of Medical Assistants

AAMC:
American Association of Medical Clinics
American Association of Medical Colleges

AAMIH: American Association for Maternal and Infant Health

AAMMC: American Association of Medical Milk Commissioners

AAMRL: American Association of Medical Record Librarians

AAO:
American Academy of Osteopathy
American Association of Orthodontists
amino acid oxidase

AAOO: American Academy of Ophthalmology and Otolaryngology

AAOP: American Academy of Oral Pathology

AAP:
American Academy of Pediatrics
American Academy of Periodontology

AAPB: American Association of Pathologists and Bacteriologists

AAPHP: American Association of Public Health Physicians

AAPMR: American Association of Physical Medicine and Rehabilitation

AAPS:
American Association of Physicians and Surgeons
American Association of Plastic Surgeons

AART: American Association for Respiratory Therapy

AAS:
anthrax antiserum
aortic arch syndrome

AATCC: American Association of Textile Chemists and Colorists

AB:
abortion
Aid to The Blind
apex beat
Artium Baccalaureus (L) Bachelor of Arts
asthmatic bronchitis
axiobuccal

A>B: air greater than bone (conduction)

AB-100: *bis* (ethyleneimido) phosphorourethane

Ab: antibody

ab:
abortion
about
antibody

ABA: abscisic acid

abbr: abbreviation(ed)

ABC:
aconite, belladonna, chloroform
antigen-binding capacity
atomic, biological, chemical (with reference to warfare)
axiobuccocervical

ABCC: Atomic Bomb Casualty Commission

ABCP: Association of Blind Chartered Physiotherapists

abd:
abdomen(inal)
abduction(or)

abdom: abdomen(inal)

ABE: acute bacterial endocarditis

ABG:
arterial blood gases
axiobuccogingival

ABL: axiobuccolingual

Abn: abnormal

abnor: abnormal

ABO: absent bed occupancy

ABOB: N^1N^1-anhydrobis (B-hydroxyethyl) biguanide hydrochloride

Abor: abortion

ABP:
androgen-binding protein
arterial blood pressure

ABR:
Abortus Bing Ringprobe (test)
absolute bed rest

ABr test: agglutination test for brucellosis

abras: abrasions

ABS:
  acrylonitrile-butadiene-styrene
  acute brain syndrome
  alkylbenzyl sulfonates

abs:
  absent
  absolute

abs feb: *absente febre* (L) in the absence of fever

abstr: abstract

abt: about

ABY: acid bismuth yeast (agar)

AC:
  acetylcholine
  acute
  adrenal cortex or corticoid
  air conduction
  alternating current
  anodal closure
  anti-inflammatory corticoid
  atriocarotid
  auriculocarotid
  axiocervical

Ac:
  accelerator (ex., *Ac-globulin*)
  acetyl
  acryl group
  actinium (chemical symbol for)

ac:
  acute
  ante cibum (L) before meals

ACA:
  American Chiropractic Association
  American College of Allergists
  American College of Anesthesiologists
  American College of Angiology
  American College of Apothecaries

acad: academy

ACC: anodal closure contraction

Acc: adenoid cystic carcinoma

acc:
  acceleration
  accident
  accommodation
  according

AcCh: acetylcholine

accid: accident(al)

ACCL: anodal closure clonus

AcCoA: acetyl coenzyme A

accom: accommodation

accur: *accuratissime* (L) most carefully, accurately

ACD:
  absolute cardiac dullness
  acid, citrate dextrose (solution)
  actinium emanation (chemical symbol for)
  anterior chest diameter

AC-DC: bisexual (homosexual and heterosexual)

ACD sol: citric acid, trisodium citrate, dextrose solution

ACE:
  adrenal cortical extract
  alcohol-chloroform-ether (mixture)
  American Council of Education

ACF: accessory clinical findings

ACFO: American College of Foot Orthopedists

ACFS: American College of Foot Surgeons

ACG:
  American College of Gastroenterology
  angiocardiography
  apex cardiogram

AcG: accelerator globulin (factor V)

ACGP: American College of General Practitioners

ACH:
  adrenal cortical hormone
  arm, chest, height

ACH index: arm girth, chest depth, hip width index (of nutrition)

ACh: acetylcholine

ACHA: American College of Hospital Administrators

AChE: acetylcholinesterase

AChS: Associate of the Society of Chiropodists

AC&HS: before meals and at bedtime

ACI: anticlonus index

acid p'tase: acid phosphatase

ACN:
  American College of Neuropsychiatrists

acute conditioned necroses

ACNM: American College of Nurse-Midwives

ACO: anodal closing odour

ACOG: American College of Obstetricians and Gynecologists

ACOHA: American College of Osteopathic Hospital Administrators

ACOI: American College of Osteopathic Internists

ACOOG: American College of Osteopathic Obstetricians and Gynecologists

ACOP: American College of Osteopathic Pediatricians

ACOS: American College of Osteopathic Surgeons

acous: acoustics(ical)

ACP:
acyl carrier protein
American College of Pathologists
American College of Physicians
Animal Care Panel
anodal closing picture
Association of Clinical Pathologists

ACPM: American College of Preventative Medicine

ACPP: adrenocorticopolypeptide

ACR:
American College of Radiology
anticonstipation regimen

Acr: acrylic

ACS:
American Cancer Society
American Chemical Society
American College of Surgeons
anodal closing sound
antireticular cytotoxic serum
aperture current setting

ACSP: Advisory Council on Scientific Policy

ACT:
achievement through counselling and treatment
anticoagulant therapy

act: active

ACTe: anodal closure tetanus

ACTH: adrenocorticotrophic hormone

ACTN: adrenocorticotrophin

ACTP: adrenocorticotrophic polypeptide

AD:
adenoid degeneration (virus)
alcohol dehydrogenase
anodal duration
antigenic determinant
auris dextra (L) right ear
average deviation
axiodistal
diphenylchlorarsine
drug addict

Ad: adrenal

ad:
adde or *addetur* (L) let them be added
axiodistal

ADA:
American Dental Association
American Diabetes Association
American Dietetic Association

ADAP: American Dental Assistant's Program

ADAMHA: Alcohol, Drug Abuse, and Mental Health Administration

ADC:
Aid to Dependent Children
albumin, dextrose, catalase (media)
anodal duration contraction
axiodistocervical

AdC: adrenal cortex

add:
adde (L) add
addantur (L) let them be added
addition
adductor(ion)

add c trit: *àdde cum tritu* (L) add triturition

ad def an: *ad defectionem animi* (L) to the point of fainting

ad deliq: *ad deliquium* (L) to fainting

addict: addiction

addn: addition

ADE: acute disseminated encephalitis

ad effect: *ad effectum* (L) until effectual

ad feb: *adstante febre* (L) fever being present

ADG: axiodistogingival
ad gr acid: *ad gratum aciditatem* (L) to an agreeable acidity
ad gr gust: *ad gratum gustum* (L) to an agreeable taste
ADH: antidiuretic hormone (vasopressin)
adhib: *adhibendus* (L) to be administered
ADI:
  acceptable daily intake
  axiodistoincisal
ad int: *ad interim* (L) meanwhile
adj:
  adjective
  adjunct
ADL: activities of daily living
ad lib: *ad libitum* (L) at pleasure
AdM: adrenal medulla
Adm: admission, admitted
Admin: administer, administration
admov: *admove, admoveatur* (L) apply, let it be applied
ADMS: Assistant Director of Medical Services
ad naus: *ad nauseam* (L) to the extent of producing nausea
ad neut: *ad neutralizandum* (L) to neutralization
 ADO: axiodisto-occlusal
ADP:
  adenosine diphosphate
  automatic data processing
ad part dolent: *ad partes dolentes* (L) to the painful parts
ADPL: average daily patient load
ad pond om: *ad pondus omnium* (L) to the weight of the whole
ADR: Accepted Dental Remedies
Adr: adrenaline
ADS:
  antidiuretic substance
  Army Dental Services
ad sat: *ad saturandum* (L) to saturation
adst feb: *adstante febre* (L) when fever is present
ADT:
  a placebo, meaning A (*any*), D (*what you desire*), T (*thing*)
  accepted dental therapeutic
  agar-gel diffusion test

  alternate-day treatment
ADTA: American Dental Trade Association
ADTe: tetanic contraction
ad us: *ad usum* (L) according to custom
ad us ext: *ad usum externum* (L) for external use
A/DV: arterio/deep venous
AD virus: adenovirus
adv: *adversum* (L) against, adverse to
ad 2 vic: *ad duas vices* (L) at two times, for two doses
A5D5W: alcohol 5%, dextrose 5%, in water
ADX: adrenalectomized
AE:
  above-elbow
  antitoxic unit (German abbreviation for)
  energy of activation
A+E: Accident and Emergency (Ward or Dept)
AEA:
  alcohol, ether, acetone (solution)
  Atomic Energy Authority
AEC:
  at earliest convenience
  Atomic Energy Commission
AEE: Atomic Energy Establishment
AEG: air encephalogram
aeg: *aegra* (L) the patient
AEP: average evoked potential
AEq: age equivalent
aeq: *aequales* (L) equal
AER:
  acoustic evoked response
  aldosterone excretion rate
AERE: Atomic Energy Research Establishment
Aero: *Aerobacter*
AES:
  American Encephalographic Society
  American Epidemiological Society
AET: 2-amino-ethyl-isothiouronium bromide
aet: *aetas* (L) age
  aetiology

aetat: *aetatis* (L) of age
aetiol: aetiology
AF:
acid-fast
Air Force
albumin-free (tuberculin)
aldehyde fuchsin
amniotic fluid
angiogenesis factor
Armed Forces
Arthritis Foundation
atrial fibrillation
audio frequency
auricular fibrillation
af: audiofrequency
AFB:
acid-fast bacillus
American foulbrood
AFDC: Aid to Families with Dependent Children
aff:
afferent
affinis (L) having an affinity with but not identical with
AFI: amaurotic familial idiocy
AFib: atrial fibrillation
AFIP: Armed Forces Institute of Pathology
AFL: anti-fatty liver (with reference to a factor in pancreatic tissue)
AFML: Armed Forces Medical Library
aFP: alpha-fetoprotein
AFQT: Armed Forces Qualification Test
AFR: ascorbic free radical
AFRD: acute febrile respiratory disease
AFRI: acute febrile respiratory illness
AFTC: apparent free testosterone concentration
AG:
antiglobulin
antigravity
atrial gallop
axiogingival
A/G ratio: albumin-globulin ratio
Ag:
antigen
silver (L) *argentum* (chemical symbol for)

AGA:
accelerated growth area
American Gastroenterological Association
American Genetics Association
American Geriatrics Association
American Goiter Association
AGCT: Army General Classification Test
AGD: agarose diffusion (method)
AGE: angle of greatest extension
AGF: angle of greatest flexion
ag feb: *aggrediente febre* (L) when the fever increases
AGG: agammaglobulinaemia
agg:
agglutination(ed)
aggregate
aggl: agglutination(ed)
agglut: agglutination(ed)
AGGS: anti gas gangrene serum
AGI: Alan Guttmacher Institute
AgI: silver iodide
agit: *agita* (L) shake, stir
agit ante sum: *agita ante sumendum* (L) shake before taking
agit vas: *agitato vase* (L) the vial being shaken
AGMK: African green monkey kidney
AGN:
acute glomerulonephritis
agnosia
AGPA: American Group Practice Association
AGS: adrenogenital syndrome
AGT: antiglobulin test
agt: agent
AGTr: adrenoglomerulotrophin
AGTT: abnormal glucose tolerance test
AGV: aniline gentian violet
AH:
abdominal hysterectomy
arterial hypertension
Ah: hypermetropic astigmatism
AHA:
American Heart Association
American Hospital Association
Area Health Authority
aspartyl-hydroxamic acid
AHA(T): Area Health Authority (Teaching)

AHD:
   autoimmune haemolytic disease
   arteriosclerotic heart disease
AHE: acute haemorrhagic encephalomyelitis
AHF:
   American Hospital Formulary
   antihaemophilic factor (factor VIII)
AHG:
   antihaemophilic globulin
   antihuman globulin
AHGS: acute herpetic gingival stomatitis
AHIP: Assisted Health Insurance Plan
AHMC: Association of Hospital Management Committees
AHN: assistant head nurse
AHP:
   acute haemorrhagic pancreatitis
   Assistant House Physician
AHR: Association for Health Records
AHS:
   American Hearing Society
   American Hospital Society
   Assistant House Surgeon
AHT: antihyaluronidase titre
AHTG: antihuman thymocytic globulin
AHTP: antihuman thymocytic plasma
AI:
   accidentally incurred
   aortic incompetence
   aortic insufficiency
   artificial insemination
   atherogenic index
   axioincisal
AIA: allyso-propylacetamide
AIBA: amino-isobutyric acid
AIBS: American Institute of Biological Sciences
AICAR: amino-imidazole-carboxamide ribonucleotide
AICF: autoimmune complement fixation
AID:
   acute infectious disease
   Agency for International Development

artificial insemination by donor (heterologous insemination)
   autoimmune disease
AIH:
   American Institute of Homeopathy
   artificial insemination by husband (homologous insemination)
AIHA:
   American Industrial Hygiene Association
   autoimmune haemolytic anaemia
AIHC: American Industrial Health Conference
AIIMS: All-India Institute of Medical Sciences
AIL: angioimmunoblastic lymphadenopathy
AIN: American Institute of Nutrition
AInsuf: aortic insufficiency
AIP:
   acute intermittent porphyria
   Anatuberculin, Petragnani's integral
AIR: amino-imidazole ribonucleotide
AIU: absolute iodine uptake
AJ: ankle jerk
AK: above knee
AK amp: above knee amputation
AL:
   adaptation level
   alignment mark (cardiography)
   axiolingual
Al: aluminium (chemical symbol for)
al: *auris laeva* (L) left ear
ALA:
   American Laryngological Association
   amino-laevulinic acid
ALa: axiolabial
Ala: alanine
ALaG: axiolabiogingival
ALaL: axiolabiolingual
alb: albumin
albus: (L) white
ALC:
   Alternative Lifestyle Checklist
   avian leukosis complex
   axiolinguocervical

alc: alcohol
ALCAR: phosphoribosyl-5-amino-imidazole-carboxamide
AlcR: alcohol rub
AlCr: aluminium crown
Ald: aldolase
aldo: aldosterone
ALG:
  antilymphocyte globulin
  axiolinguogingival
alk: alkaline
alk p'tase: alkaline phosphatase
ALL: acute lymphocytic leukaemia
ALMA: Adoptee's Liberty Movement Association
ALMI: anterior lateral myocardial infarct
ALO: axiolinguo-occlusal
ALP: anterior lobe of pituitary
ALROS: American Laryngological, Rhinological, and Otological Society
ALS:
  amyotrophic lateral sclerosis
  antilymphocytic serum
ALT:
  alternate
  altitude
ALTB: acute laryngo-tracheobronchitis
alt dieb: *alternis diebus* (L) every other day
alt hor: *alternis horis* (L) every other hour
alt noc: *alternis nocta* (L) every other night
alv: alveolar
alv adst: *alvo adstricta* (L) when the bowels are constipated
alv deject: *alvi dejectiones* (L) discharge from the bowels
Alvx: alveolectomy
ALW: arch-loop-whorl
AM:
  actomyosin
  aerospace medicine
  ammeter
  amperemeter
  amplitude modulation
  anovular menstruation
  ante meridiem (L) before noon,
    in the morning
  arousal mechanism
  Artium Magister (L) Master of Arts
  aviation medicine
  axiomesial
  meter-angle
AM:
  American
  americium (chemical symbol for)
  amyl
am:
  ametropia
  meter-angle
  myopic astigmatism
AMA:
  against medical advice
  American Medical Association
  Australian Medical Association
AMAL: Aero-Medical Acceleration Laboratory
amb:
  ambulance
  ambulatory
ambig: ambiguous
ambul: ambulation (ory)
AMC:
  arthrogryposis multiplex congenita
  axiomesiocervical
AMD: axiomesiodistal
AMDS: Association of Military Dental Surgeons
AMEL: Aero-Medical Equipment Laboratory
Amer: American
AMG: axiomesiogingival
AMH: automated medical history
Amh: mixed astigmatism with myopia predominating
AMI:
  acute myocardial infarction
  Association of Medical Illustrators
  axiomesio-incisal
AML: acute myoblastic leukaemia
ammon: ammonia
AMO: axiomesio-occlusal
AMOL: acute monocytic leukaemia
amor: amorphous
amorph: amorphous

AMP:
adenosine monophosphate
amphetamine
average mean pressure
amp
ampere, amperage
amplification
ampoule
amputation
amph: amphoric
ampl: *amplus* (L) large
ampul: *ampulla* (L) ampul,
ampoule
AMR: alternating motion reflexes
AMRL: Aerospace Medical
Research Laboratories
AMS:
American Microscopical
Society
Army Medical Service
Association of Military Surgeons
auditory memory span
AMSC: Army Medical Specialist
Corps
AMT: amphetamines
amt: amount
amu: atomic mass unit
An:
actinon (chemical symbol for)
anisometropia (eyes requiring
different refractive correc-
tions)
anode(al)
A$_n$: normal atmosphere
ANA:
American Neurological
Association
American Nurses' Association
anaesthesia(ic)
antinuclear antibody
Anaes[th]: anaesthesia(ic)
anal:
analgesic
analysis(se)
Anal Psychol: analytical psy-
chology
ANAP: agglutination negative,
absorption positive
Anat: anatomy(ical)
ANC: Army Nurse Corps
AnCC: anodal closure contraction
ANDRO: androsterone
AnDTe: anodal duration tetanus

Anesth: anesthetic
an ex: anode excitation
ANF:
American Nurses' Foundation
antinuclear factors
Ang:
angiogram
angle, especially angle of
scapula
anh: anhydrous
ANIT: alpha-naphthyl-
isothiocyanate
Ann: annals
AnOC: anodal opening contraction
ANP: A-norprogesterone
ANRL: antihypertensive neutral
renomedullary lipids
ANS: autonomic nervous system
ans: answer
ANSI: American National Standards Institute (formerly ASA,
USASI)
ANT: 2-amino-5-nitro-thiazol
(Enheptin)
ant: anterior
antag: antagonistic
ant ax line: anterior axillary line
ante: *ante* (L) before
Anthrop: anthropology
anthropom: anthropometry
ant jentac: *ante jentaculum* (L)
before breakfast
Ant pit: anterior pituitary (anterior
lobe of pituitary)
Ant sup spine: anterior superior
spine (of ilium)
ANTU: alphanapthylthiourea
ANUG: acute necrotizing ulcerative gingivitis
AO:
acridine orange (test)
anodal opening
atomic orbital (contour)
AOA:
American Optometric Association
American Orthopedic Association
American Orthopsychiatric
Association
American Osteopathic Association

AOB: alcohol on breath
AOAC: Association of Official Agricultural Chemists
AOAS: American Osteopathic Academy of Sclerotherapy
AOC: anodal opening contraction
AOCA: American Osteopathic College of Anesthesiologists
AOCD: American Osteopathic College of Dermatology
AOCl: anodal opening clonus
AOCPA: American Osteopathic College of Pathologists
AOCPR: American Osteopathic College of Proctology
AOCR: American Osteopathic College of Radiology
AOCRM: American Osteopathic College of Rehabilitation
AOD: arterial occlusive desease
AOL: acro-osteolysis
AOM: Master of Obstetric Art
AOO: anodal opening odour
AOP: anodal opening picture
AOPA: American Orthotic and Prosthetics Association
Aort regurg: aortic regurgitation
Aort sten: aortic stenosis
AOS:
American Otological Society
anodal opening sound
AOT: Association of Occupational Therapists
AOTA: American Occupational Therapy Association
AOTe: anodal opening tetanus
AP:
action potential
alkaline phosphatase
alum precipitated (with reference to vaccines)
anterior pituitary
anteroposterior
aortic pressure
appendectomy
arithmetic progression
artificial pneumothorax
axiopulpal
3-AP: 3-acetylpyridine
A&P: auscultation and percussion
AP: apothecary
ap: *ante prandium* (L) before dinner

$A_2 > P_2$: aortic second sound greater than pulmonary second sound
$A_2 < P_2$: aortic second sound less than pulmonary second sound
APA:
American Pharmaceutical Association
American Physiotherapy Association
American Psychiatric Association
American Psychoanalytic Association
American Psychological Association
American Psychopathological Association
6-APA: 6-amino penicillanic acid
APAF: antipernicious anaemia factor
APC:
antiphlogistic corticoid
aperture current
aspirin, phenacetin, and caffeine
atrial premature contractions
APC virus: adenoidal, pharyngeal, conjunctival virus
APD: action potential duration
A-PD: anteroposterior diameter
APE:
acetone powder extract
anterior pituitary hormone
APHA:
American Protestant Hospital Association
American Public Health Association
APhA: American Pharmaceutical Association
APIM: Association Professionelle Internationale des Médecins
APL: anterior-pituitary-like substance
AP& Lat: anteroposterior and lateral
APM:
Academy of Physical Medicine
Academy of Psychosomatic Medicine

APMR: Association for Physical and Mental Rehabilitation

apoth: apothecary

APP: avian pancreatic polypeptide

app:
  apparent
  appendix

appar:
  apparatus
  apparent

appl:
  appliance
  applied

applan: *applanatus* (L) flattened

applicand: *applicandus* (L) to be applied

appr: approximate(ly)

approx: approximate(ly)

appt: appointment

APR: anterior pituitary reaction

aprax: apraxia

APRL: American Prosthetic Research Laboratory

APS:
  adenosine phosphosulphate
  American Pediatric Society
  American Proctologic Society
  American Psychological Society
  American Psychological Society
  American Psychosomatic Society

APT: alum-precipitated toxoid

APTA: American Physical Therapy Association

APTD: Aid to Permanently and Totally Disabled

APTT: activated partial thromboplastin time

APUD: amine precursor uptake and decarboxylation (cells)

AQ: accomplishment or achievement quotient

aq:
  aqua (L) water
  aqueous

aq astr: *aqua astricta* (L) frozen water

aq bull: *aqua bulliens* (L) boiling water

aq comm: *aqua communis* (L) common water

aq dest: *aqua destillata* (L) distilled water

aq ferv: *aqua fervens* (L) hot water

aq fluv: *aqua fluvialis* (L) river water

aq font: *aqua fontana* (L) spring water

aq mar: *aqua marina* (L) sea water

aq niv: *aqua nivalis* (L) snow water

aq pluv: *aqua pluvialis* (L) rain water

aq pur: *aqua pura* (L) pure water

aq tep: *aqua tepida* (L) lukewarm water

aqu: aqueous

AR:
  achievement ratio
  active resistive (exercise)
  alarm reaction
  analytical reagent
  apical-radial (pulse)
  arsphenamine
  articulare (craniometric point)
  atrophic rhinitis (of swine)

A/R: apical/radial

Ar: argon (chemical symbol for)

ara-A: adenine arabinoside (vidarabine)

ara-C: cyctosine arabinoside (cytarabine)

ARBOR: arthropod-borne (virus)

ARC:
  American Red Cross
  anomalous retinal correspondence

Arch: archives

ARCS: Associate of the Royal College of Science

ARD:
  absolute reaction of degeneration
  acute respiratory disease

ARDC: Air Research and Development Command

ARDS: acute respiratory distress syndrome

ARF: acute rheumatic fever

Arg: arginine

arg: *argentum* (L) silver

ARIC: Associate of the Royal Institute of Chemistry

ARM: artificial rupture of the membranes

ARMH: Academy of Religion and Mental Health

ARNMD: Association for Research in Nervous and Mental Diseases

ARO: Associate for Research in Ophthalmology

ARP:
absolute refractory period
Advanced Research Projects
American Registry of Pathologists

ARPT: American Registry of Physical Therapists

ARRC: Associate of the Royal Red Cross

ARRS: American Roentgen Ray Society

ARRT: American Registered Respiratory Therapist

ARS:
American Radium Society
American Rhinologic Society

Ars: arsphenamine

ARSPH: Associate of the Royal Society for the Promotion of Health

ART: Accredited Record Technician

art:
artery(ial)
articulation

artic: articulation

artif: artificial

art insem: artificial insemination

AS:
ankylosing spondylitis
anxiety state
aortic stenosis
aqueous solution
aqueous suspension
arteriosclerosis
auris sinistra (L) left ear

A-S: ascendance-submission

As:
arsenic (chemical symbol for)
astigmatism

ASA:
American Society of Anesthesiologists
American Standards Association
aspirin (acetylsalicylic acid)

ASAIO: American Society for Artificial Internal Organs

ASAP: as soon as possible

ASB: American Society of Bacteriology

ASC: acetylsulphanilyl chloride

asc:
arteriosclerosis(tic)
ascending

ASCH: American Society of Clinical Hypnosis

ASCLT: American Society of Clinical Laboratory Technicians

ASCP: American Society of Clinical Pathologists

ascr: *ascriptum* (L) ascribed to

ASCVD: arteriosclerotic cardiovascular disease

ASD: atrial septal defect

ASDR: American Society of Dental Radiographers

ASE: axilla, shoulder, elbow (bandage)

ASF: alinine, sulphur and formaldehyde (microscopy)

ASG: American Society for Genetics

ASGB: Anatomical Society of Great Britain and Ireland

ASH: American Society for Hematology

AsH: hypertrophic astigmatism

ASHA:
American School Health Association
American Speech and Hearing Association

ASHBM: Associate Scottish Hospital Bureau of Management

ASHD: arteriosclerotic heart disease

ASHI: Association for Study of Human Infertility

ASHP: American Society of Hospital Pharmacists

ASII: American Science Information Institute

ASIM: American Society of Internal Medicine

ASL: antistreptolysin titre

ASLIB: Association of Special Libraries and Information Bureaux

ASLO: antistreptolysin-O

AsM: myopic astigmatism

ASME: Association for the Study of Medical Education
ASMT: American Society of Medical Technologists
Asn: asparagine
ASO:
American Society of Orthodontists
antistreptolysin-O
ASOS: American Society of Oral Surgeons
ASP: American Society of Parasitologists
Asp: aspartic acid
ASR: aldosterone secretion rate
ASRT: American Society of Radiologic Technologists
ASS: anterior superior spine
Assn: association
assocd: associated (with)
asst: assistant
Ast: astigmatism
ASTEC: Association of Science Technology Centers
A sten: aortic stenosis
Asth: asthenopia
ASTHO: Association of State and Territorial Health Officials
ASTI: antispasticity index
ASTM: American Society for Testing and Materials
ASTMH: American Society of Tropical Medicine and Hygiene
ASTO: antistreptolysin-O
As tol: as tolerated
A/SV: arterio/superficial venous
asym: asymmetrical
AT:
achievement test
adjunctive therapy
air temperature
alt Tuberculin (Ger) old tuberculin
AT$_7$: hexachlorophene
AT$_{10}$: dihydrotachysterol
At: astatine (chemical symbol for)
at:
airtight
atom(ic)
ATA: alimentary toxic aleukia
ATCC: American Type Culture Collection

at fib: atrial fibrillation
ATG: antithrombocyte globulin
ATH: acetyl-tyrosine hydrazide
ATHC: allotetrahydrocortisol
Athsc: atherosclerosis
ATL: Achilles tendon lengthening
ATLAS: an electronic digital computer
atm: atmosphere(ic)
atmos: atmosphere(ic)
at no: atomic number
ATP: adenosine triphosphate
ATPase: adenosine triphosphatase
ATPD: ambient temperature and pressure, dry
ATPS: ambient temperature and pressure, saturated
ATR: Achilles tendon reflex
atr: atrophy
ATS:
American Trudeau Society
antitetanic serum
anxiety tension state
att: attending
AT type: adenine and thymine type (with reference to pentosenucleic acids)
at wt: atomic weight
AU:
Ångstrom unit
antitoxin unit (diphtheria)
aures unitas (L) both ears (together)
auris uterque (L) each ear
Australia (antigen)
Au: gold (L) *aurum* (chemical symbol for)
[198]**AU:** radioactive gold (chemical symbol for)
auct: *auctorum* (L) of authors
aud: auditory
aur fib: auricular fibrillation
auric: auricular
AuSh: Australian serum hepatitis
aux: auxiliary
AV:
anteversion (ed)
aortic valve
arteriovenous
atrioventricular
auriculoventricular
average

avoirdupois
AVA: arteriovenous anastomosis
AVC:
allantoid vaginal cream
atrioventricular canal
avdp: avoirdupois
AVI: air velocity index
AVMA: American Veterinary Medical Association
AVN: atrioventricular node
AVP: antiviral protein
AVS: Association for Voluntary Sterilization
AVT: arginine vasotonin
AW:
above waist
atomic warfare
A & W: alive and well
AWF: adrenal weight factor (a corticotrophin in ACTH)
ax:
axilla (ary)
axis(ial)
ax grad: axial gradient
AXM: acetoxycyclo-hexamine (a catecholamine)
Az: azote (nitrogen)
AZT: Aschheim-Zondek test (for pregnancy)

B

B:
Bacillus
balneum (L) bath
barometric
base (in chemical formulas)
base (of prism)
bath
Baumé scale
behaviour
Benoist scale
benzoate
bicuspid
blue
body (in psychology, all the body except nervous system)
bone-marrow derived (lymphocytes)
boron (chemical symbol for)
brother
buccal

bursa cells (of thymus or lymph nodes)
b:
bis (L) twice, two times
boils at (when followed by a figure designating degrees)
born
β:
beta (second letter of Greek alphabet)
In chemistry, in organic compounds, it refers to the carbon atom next to the carbon atom bearing the active group of molecules
Symbol designating *second*
BA:
Bachelor of Arts
backache
balneum arenae (L) sand bath
basion (craniometric point)
Biological Abstracts
blood agar
boric acid
bronchial asthma
buccoaxial
B>A: bone greater than air
Ba: barium (chemical symbol for)
BAA: benzoyl arginine amide
Bab: Babinski (reflex)
BAC:
bacterial antigen complex
blood alcohol concentration
British Association of Chemists
buccoaxiocervical
Bact: *Bacterium*
bact:
bacteria(al)
bacteriology
BAD: British Association of Dermatology
BaE: barium enema
Ba enem: barium enema
BAG: buccoaxiogingival
BAGG: buffered azide glucose glycerol (broth)
BAL: British anti-lewisite (2, 3, dimercaptopropanol)
bal:
balance(d)
balsam
bal arenae: *balneum arenae* (L) sand bath

bal mar: *balneum maris* (L) salt or sea-water bath
bal vap: *balneum vapour* (L) steam or vapour bath
BaM: barium meal
BAN: British Association of Neurologists
BAO:
Bachelor of the Art of Obstetrics
basal acid output
British Association of Otolaryngologists
BAP:
blood agar plate
brachial artery pressure
BAPhysMed: British Association of Physical Medicine
BAPS:
British Association of Paediatric Surgeons
British Association of Plastic Surgeons
BAPT: British Association of Physical Training
bar: barometer(ric)
BAS: benzyl analogue of serotonin
bas: basophil(s)
BASH: body acceleration synchronous with heart beat
basos: basophils
BAUS: British Association of Urological Surgeons
BB:
bed bath
blanket bath
blood bank
both bones (with reference to fractures)
breakthrough bleeding
breast biopsy
BBA: born before arrival
BBB:
blood-brain barrier
bundle-branch block
BBC: brombenzylcyanide (a war gas)
BBT: basal body temperature
BC:
Bachelor of Surgery
birth control
Blue Cross
bone conduction

buccocervical
BCA: Blue Cross Association
BCB: brilliant cresyl blue
BC/BS: Blue Cross/Blue Shield
BCC: Birth Control Clinic
BCCG: British Co-operative Clinical Group
BCE: basal cell epithelioma
BCG:
bacille Calmette-Guérin
ballistocardiogram
bromcresyl green (an indicator)
BCG test: bicolour guaiac test
BCH: basal cell hyperplasia
BCh: Bachelor of Surgery
BChD: Bachelor of Dental Surgery
BCIC: Birth Control Investigation Committee
BCM: birth control medication
BCME: bis chlormethyl ether
BCNU: 1, 3 bis 2-chlorethyl-nitrosourea
BCP: bromcresyl purple
BCS: British Cardiac Society
BCTF: Breast Cancer Task Force (NCI)
BCW: Biological and Chemical Warfare
BD:
base deficit
base of prism down
bile duct
borderline dull
buccodistal
B&D: bondage and discipline
Bd: board
bd: *bis die* (L) twice a day
BDA: British Dental Association
BDAC: Bureau of Drug Abuse Control
BDB: bis-diazotized-benzidine
BDC: burn-dressing change
BDE: bile duct examination
BDentSci: Bachelor of Dental Science (Dublin)
BDG: buffered desoxycholate glucose (broth)
BDH: British Drug Houses (Research, Inc)
BDS:
Bachelor of Dental Surgery
biological detection system
BDSc: Bachelor of Dental Science

BE:
  Bacillen Emulsion (Ger.)
  barium enema
  base excess
  below elbow
  bile esculin
  broncho-esophagology
Be: beryllium (chemical
  symbol for)
Bé: Beaumé (specific gravity
  scale)
BEAR: Biological Effects of
  Atomic Radiation (Com-
  mittee)
beg: begin
beh: behaviour(ism)
BEI: butanol-extractable iodine
ben: *bene* (L) well, good
Benz: benzidine
BES: balanced electrolyte solution
bet: between
beV: billion electron volts
BF:
  bentonite flocculation (test)
  blastogenic factor
  bouillon filtre (Fr.) bouillon filtrate tuberculin; Denys' tuberculin)
  breakfast fed
  buffered
  butter fat
B/F: bound/free (antigens)
BFP: biological false positive
BFR sol: buffered Ringer's solution
BG:
  bicolor guaiac (test)
  blood glucose
  buccogingival
B-G: Bordet-Gengou (bacillus)
BGE: butyl glycidyl ether
BGG: bovine gamma globulin
BGGRA: British Gelatine and Glue
  Research Association
BGLB: brilliant green lactose broth
BGS: British Geriatrics Society
BH:
  bill of health
  brain hormone
BHC: benzene hexachloride (an
  insecticide and scabicide)
BHI: Bureau of Health Insurance
BHIB: beef heart infusion broth

BHIS: beef heart infusion sup-
  plemented (broth or agar)
BHL: biological half-life
BHM: Bureau of Health Manpower
BHN: bephenium hydroxy-
  naphthoate
BHPRD: Bureau of Health Planning and Resources
  Development
BHyg: Bachelor of Hygiene
BI:
  base of prism in
  bone injury
Bi: bismuth (chemical symbol for)
BIAC: Bioinstrumentation Advisory Council
bib: *bibe* (L) drink
biblio: bibliography
BIBRA: British Industrial Biological Research Association
bicarb: bicarbonate
BID: brought in dead
bid: *bis in die* (L) twice a day
BIH: benign intracranial hypertension
bihor: *bihorium* (L) during two
  hours
Bi Isch: between ischial
  tuberosities
BIL: bilirubin (test)
bilat: bilateral
bili, bilirub: bilirubin
bin: *bis in noctus* (L) twice a night
Biochem: biochemistry(ical)
Biol: biology(ical)
Biophys: biophysics
BIOS: British Intelligence Objective Subcommittee
BIP:
  bacterial intravenous protein
  biparietal diameter (of skull)
  bismuth iodoform paraffin
BIPM: *Bureau International des
  Poids et Mesures* (Inter-
  national Bureau of Weights
  and Measures)
BIPP: bismuth iodoform petrol-
  atum paste
BIR:
  basic incidence rate
  British Institute of Radiology
BiSP: between ischial spines
BiT: between great trochanters

BITU: benzyl-thiourea
BJ:
  Bence Jones (protein)
  biceps jerk
B&J: bone and joint
BJM: bones, joints, muscles
BK: below knee (with reference to amputation stump)
Bk: berkelium (chemical symbol for)
BKA: below the knee amputation
bkf: breakfast
BKTT: below knee to toe
BKWP: below knee walking plaster
BL:
  buccolingual
  Burkitt's lymphoma
Bl: black
bl:
  bleeding
  blood
  blue
B-l: bursa equivalent lymphocyte
BLB mask: Boothby-Lovelace-Bulbulian mask (for oxygen administration)
Bl C: blood culture
bl cult: blood culture
BLG: beta-lactoglobulin
BIP: blood pressure
BLOT: British Library of Tape (Recordings)
BLROA: British Laryngological, Rhinological and Otological Association
Bl S: blood sugar
Bl T: blood type
BM:
  Bachelor of Medicine
  basal metabolism
  bowel movement
  buccomesial
bm: *balneum maris* (L) sea-water bath
BMA: British Medical Association
BMB: British Medical Bulletin
BME: basal medium, Eagle's
BMPP: benign mucous membrane pemphigus
BMR: basal metabolic rate
BMS: Bachelor of Medical Science

BMSA: British Medical Students Association
BMSJ: British Medical Students Journal
BNA: Basle (Basel) Nomina Anatomica
BNDD: Bureau of Narcotics and Dangerous Drugs
BNF: British National Formulary
BNO: bowels not opened
BO:
  base of prism out
  body odour
  Bolton (craniometric point)
  bowels open
  bucco-occlusal
Bo: bohemium (now called rhenium) (chemical symbol for)
bo: bowel
B&O: belladonna and opium
BOA:
  born on arrival
  British Orthopaedic Association
BOD: biochemical oxygen demand
BodUnits: Bodansky units (with reference to alkaline phosphatase)
BOEA: ethyl biscoumacetate
boil: boiling
bol: *bolus* (L) a large pill
BOP: Buffalo orphan prototype (with reference to viruses)
BOR: bowels open regularly
Bot: botany, botanical
bot: bottle
BOW: bag of waters (amniotic sac)
BP:
  barometric pressure
  bathroom privileges
  bed pan
  biotic potential
  biparietal (diameter of head)
  birth place
  blood pressure
  British Pharmacopoeia
  buccopulpal
  bypass
bp: boiling point
BPA: British Paediatric Association
BPB: bromophenol blue

BPC: British Pharmaceutical Codex
BPH: benign prostatic hypertrophy
B Ph: British Pharmacopoeia
BPharm: Bachelor of Pharmacy
BPL: B-propriolactone
BP 120/80 lar: blood pressure 120 (systolic), 80 (diastolic), left arm reclining or recumbent
BPMF: British Postgraduate Medical Federation
BPP: bovine pancreatic polypeptide
BPV: bovine papilloma virus
BP(Vet): British Pharmacopoeia (veterinary)
BQC sol: 2, 6-dibromoquinonechlorimide solution
BR:
 bathroom
 bed rest
 British Revision of BNA (with reference to anatomical nomenclature)
Br:
 bridge (dentistry)
 bromine (chemical symbol for)
 bronchitis
 brown
 Brucella
br:
 boiling range
 branch
 breath
 brother
BRCS: British Red Cross Society
Brhp: bronchophony
BRI: Bio-Research Index
Brit: British
Brkf: breakfast
BRL: Beecham Research Laboratories
BRO: bronchoscopy
Bron: bronchial
Bronch: bronchoscopist-(oscopy)(ic)
BRP: bathroom privileges
BRS: British Roentgen Society
Br sounds: breath sounds
BS:
 Bachelor of Science
 Bachelor of Surgery
 blood sugar

 Blue Shield
 bowel sound
 breath sound
 British Standard
 Bureau of Standards
BSA:
 benzenesulphonic acid
 body surface area
 bovine serum albumin
BSc: Bachelor of Science
BSCC: British Society for Clinical Cytology
BSE: breast self-examination
B&S glands: Bartholin's and Skene's glands
BSI: British Standards Institution
BSL: blood sugar level
BSN:
 Bachelor of Science in Nursing
 bowel sounds normal
BSP: bromsulphalein
BSp: bronchospasm
BSR: blood sedimentation rate
BSS: buffered salt (saline) solution
BST:
 blood serological test
 brief stimulus therapy (psychology)
BT:
 bedtime
 bitemporal (diameter of head)
 blue tetrazolium (a histological stain)
 body temperature
 brain tumour
BTA: N-benzoyl-l-tyrosine amide
BTB:
 breakthrough bleeding
 bromthymol blue (an indicator)
BThU: British Thermal Unit
BTPS: body temperature, pressure (prevailing atmospheric), and saturation (water vapour)
BTS: Blood Transfusion Service
BTU: British thermal unit
BTX: benzene, toluene, xylene
BU:
 base of prism up
 Bodansky units
 bromouracil
 Burn Unit
Bu: butyl

Bucc: buccal
BUDU: bromodeoxyuridine
bull:
  bulletin
  bulliat (L) let it boil
BuMed: Bureau of Medicine and Surgery, U.S. Navy
BUN: blood urea nitrogen
BUPA: British United Provident Association
bur: bureau
Burd: Burdick suction
But: *butyrum* (L) butter
BV:
  biological value
  blood vessel
  blood volume
bv: *balneum vaporis* (L) vapour bath
BVA: British Veterinary Association
BVM: bronchovascular markings
BVSc: Bachelor of Veterinary Science
BW:
  below waist
  biological warfare
  birth weight
  blood Wassermann
  body water
  body weight
BWD: bacillary white diarrhoea (in chicks)
BX: biopsy
BYE: Barile-Yaguchi-Eveland (medium)
BZ: benzoyl

C

C:
  A symbol for any *constant*
  calorie (large)
  canine tooth (permanent)
  carbon (chemical symbol for)
  carrier
  cathode
  Roman Catholic
  Celsius scale or thermometer
  centigrade (temperature scale)
  central
  certified
  cervical
  chest (precordial) lead (in electro-cardiography)
  clearance (renal)
  clonus
  closure
  coarse (with reference to bacterial colonies)
  cocaine
  coefficient
  coloured
  colour sense
  complement
  complete
  compliance
  concentration
  congius (L) gallon
  contraction
  control (with reference to a group in an experiment)
  cortex
  costa (rib)
  coulomb
  crystalline enzyme
  cylinder
  cytidine
  cytochrome
  cytosine
c:
  calorie (small)
  candle
  canine tooth (deciduous)
  capacity
  centi (prefix)
  centum (L) one hundred
  cibus (L) meal
  circa (L) about
  contact
  cubic
  cum (L) with
  curie
  cyclic
c̄: with
C': complement (bacteriology)
C1, C2, C3 (etc): cervical nerves or cervical vertebrae No. 1, No. 2, No. 3 (etc)
CI, CII, CIII, (etc): cranial nerves I, II, etc.
C_1, C_2, C_3: costa (rib) I (first rib), etc

C_1, C_2, C_3: cytochromes 1, 2, and 3

C_1 to C_9: components of complement

C_3: Collin's solution (for perfusion)

C-6: hexamethonium (Vegolysin)

C-10: decamethonium

^{137}C: radioactive caesium

^{14}C: radioactive carbon

C_{alb}: albumin clearance

C_{cr}: creatinine clearance

C_{in}: inulin clearance

C_p: phosphate clearance

C_{pah}: p-aminohippurate clearance

C_{T-1824}: clearance of Evans blue

CA:
  carbonic anhydrase
  carcinoma (cancer)
  cardiac arrest
  cervicoaxial
  Chemical Abstracts
  chronological age
  cold agglutination (test)
  common antigen
  coronary artery
  corpora alata (endocrinology)
  cortisone acetate
  Council Accepted (American Medical Association)
  croup-associated (virus)
  cytosine arabinoside

Ca:
  calcium (chemical symbol for)
  carcinoma (cancer)
  cathode (al)

ca:
  candle
  circa (L) about (with reference to time)

CAAT: computer-assisted axial tomography

CAC: cardiac-accelerator centre

CaCC: cathodal closure contraction

CACX: cancer of the cervix

CAD: coronary artery desease

CaDTe: cathodal duration tetanus

CAE: contingent after-effects

CaEDTA:
  calcium disodium ethylene diamine tetra-acetate
  edathamil calcium disodium

caerul: caeruleus (L) dark blue, dark green

caf: caffeine

CAG: chronic atrophic gastritis

CAH: cyanacetic acid hydrazine

CAI:
  computer-aided instruction
  confused artificial insemination

CAL: calcium test (dentistry)

Cal: calorie, large

cal:
  calibre
  calorie, small

calCd: calculated

calef: calefactus (L) warmed; or calefac (L) make warm

CAM: chorio-allantoic membrane

CAMP: Christie, Atkins, Munch-Peterson (test)

cAMP: cyclic adenosine monophosphate

canc: cancelled

CAO: chronic airway obstruction

CáOC: cathodal opening contraction

CAP:
  chloramphenicol
  College of American Pathologists
  Community Action Program
  cystine aminopeptidase

cap:
  capacity
  capiat (L) let him take
  capsula (L) capsule

cap moll: capsula mollis (L) soft capsule

cap quant vult: capiat quantum vult (L) let the patient take as much as he will

caps: capsule (L) capsule

CAR: Canadian Association of Radiologists

carb: carbonate

carbo: carbohydrate

Cardiol: cardiology

CARF: Commission on Accreditation and Rehabilitation Facilities

CAS:
  Chemical Abstracts Service
  control adjustment strap
  Council of Academic Societies

Cas: casualty
CASHD: coronary arteriosclerotic heart disease
CAST: Clearinghouse Announcements in Science and Technology
CAT: .
catecholamines
child's apperception test
college ability test
computerized axial tomography
Cath: Catholic
cath:
cathartic
catheter(ize)
Cau: Caucasian
Caud: caudal
CAV:
congenital absence of vagina
congenital adrenal virilism
cav: cavity
CAVD: In psychology, a battery of four tests of intelligence (completion, arithmetic problems, vocabulary, following directions)
CA virus: croup-associated virus
CB:
carbobenzoxy
chest-back
Chirurgiae Baccalaureus (L) Bachelor of Surgery
chronic bronchitis
CB$_{11}$: phenadoxine
Cb: columbium (chemical symbol) (SEE *Nb*)
CBA: chronic bronchitis and asthma
CBC: complete blood count
CBD:
closed bladder drainage
common bile duct
CBF: cerebral blood flow
CBG: corticosteroid-binding globulin (transcortin)
CBI: close-binding-intimate
CBN: Commission on Biological Nomenclature
CBR:
chemical, biological, and radiological (warfare)
complete bed rest

crude birth rate
CBS: chronic brain syndrome
CBW:
chemical, biological warfare
critical band width (of noise)
CBz: carbobenzoxychloride
CC:
chief complaint
classical conditioning
coefficient of correlation
commission certified (with reference to stains)
computer calculated
corpora cardiaca (endocrinology)
critical condition
current complaints
Cc: concave
cc:
cubic centimetre
with correction (ophthalmology)
CCA:
cephalin cholesterol antigen
chick cell agglutination (unit)
chimpanzee coryza agent
C-C-A: cytidyl-cytidyl-adenyl
CCAT: conglutinating complement absorption test
CCBV: central circulating blood volume
CCC:
calcium cyanamide (carbimide) citrated
cathodal closure contraction
CCCl: cathodal closure clonus
CCCR: closed chest cardiac resuscitation
CCD: calibration curve data
CCDN: Central Council for District Nursing
CCF: congestive cardiac failure
CCHE: Central Council for Health Education
CCI: chronic coronary insufficiency
CCK: cholecystokinin
CCME: Coordinating Council of Medical Education
CCMS: clean catch midstream
CCMT: catechol-O-methyl transferase
CCS: casualty clearing station

CCT:
chocolate-coated tablet
coated compressed tablet
controlled cord traction
CCTe: cathodal closure tetanus
CCU: Coronary Care Unit
CCW: counter clockwise
CD:
cadaver donor
Caesarean delivered
canine distemper
canine dose
cardiovascular disease
Carrel-Dakin (fluid)
civil defence
colla destra (L) with the right
hand
communicable disease
completely denatured
conjugata diagonalis (L)
diagonal conjugate (diameter
of pelvic inlet)
contact dermatitis
convulsive disorder
convulsive dose
curative dose
cystic duct
Cd:
cadmium (chemical symbol for)
caudal or coccygeal, with reference to vertebrae
cd: candela
CD$_{50}$: median curative dose (that
which abolishes symptoms in
50% of test subjects)
^{115}**Cd:** radioactive cadmium
CDAA: chloro-diallylacetamide, a
herbicide
C&DB: cough and deep-breathe
CDC:
calculated date of confinement
Center for Disease Control (formerly Communicable Dis-
ease Center of HEW,
Atlanta)
CDE: canine distemper
encephalitis
CDP: cytidine diphosphate
CDPC: cytidine diphosphate
choline
CDT:
carbon dioxide therapy
Certified Dental Technician

CE:
cardiac enlargement
chemical energy
chick embryo
constant error
contractile element (of skeletal
muscle)
cytopathic effect
Ce: cerium (chemical symbol for)
^{58}**Ce:** radioactive cerium
C/E: Church of England
C-E mixture: chloroform-ether
mixture
CEA: carcinoembryonic antigen
CEFMG: Council on Education for
Foreign Medical Graduates
cej: cement-enamel junction
Cel: Celsius (thermometric scale)
cell: celluloid (dentistry)
CELO: chicken embryo lethal
orphan (virus)
CEM: conventional-transmission
electron microscope
cen: central
cent:
centigrade
central
CEO: chick embryo origin
CEP: countercurrent electro-
phoresis
CEPA: chloroethane phosphoric
acid
ceph-floc: cephalin flocculation
(test)
CEQ: Council on Environmental
Quality
CER: conditioned emotional
response
CERN: Conseil Européen de
Recherche Nucleaire
(Geneva)
cert:
certificate
certified
cerv: cervical, cervix
CES: central excitatory state
CETI: Communication with
Extraterrestrial Intelligence
CF:
cancer-free
carbolfuchsin
cardiac failure
Carworth Farms

chest and left leg lead
Christmas factor (PTC)
citrovorum factor (folinic acid)
colicin factor
complement fixation
coronary flow
counting fingers
cystic fibrosis
Cf: californium (chemical symbol for)
cf: *confer* (L) compare with or refer to
c/f: coloured female
CFA: complete Freund's adjunct
C-factor: cleverness factor (psychology)
CFF: critical fusion or flicker frequency
CFI: complement fixation inhibition (test)
CFM: chlorofluromethane (flurocarbon)
cfm: cubic feet per minute
CFMG: Commission on Foreign Medical Graduates
cfs: cubic feet per second
CFSE: crystal field stabilization energy
CFSTI: Clearinghouse for Federal and Technical Information (later NTIS)
CFT: complement-fixation test
CFU: colony-forming unit
CFW: Carworth Farm mice (Webster strain)
CG:
choking gas (phosgene)
chorionic gonadotrophin
control group
iodocyanine green
phosgene
cg:
centigram
centre of gravity
CGD: chronic granulomatous disease
CGH: chorionic gonadotrophic hormone
CGI: carbimazole
CGM: central grey matter (of spinal cord)
cgm: centigram
CGN: chronic glomerulonephritis

CGP:
N-carbobenzoxy-glycyl-L-phenylalanine
chorionic growth-hormone prolactin
circulating granulocyte pool
CGS: catgut suture
CGS unit: centimetre-gram second unit
CGT: N-carbobenzoxy-α-glutamyl-L-tyrosine
CH: crown-heel (with reference to length of fetus)
CH: Christchurch chromosome
C&H: cocaine and heroin
Ch:
chapter
check
chest
chief
child
choline
cH: hydrogen ion concentration
CHA:
Catholic Hospital Association
congenital hypoplastic anaemia
ChA: choline acetylase
chap: chapter
chart: *charta* (L) a paper
chart bib: *charta bibula* (L) blotting paper
chart cerat: *charta cerata* (L) waxed paper
CHB: complete heart block
ChB: *Chirurgiae Baccalaureus* (L) Bachelor of Surgery
CHC:
Community Health Center
Community Health Council
CHD:
Chediak-Higashi disease
childhood disease
coronary heart disease
ChD: *Chirurgiae Doctor* (L) Doctor of Surgery
ChE: cholinesterase
chem: chemistry(ical)
CHF: congestive heart failure
chg: change
Chir Doct: *Chirurgiae Doctor* (L) Doctor of Surgery
Chl: chloroform
Chlb: chlorobutanol

ChM: *Chirurgiae Magister* (L) Master of Surgery

CHIP: Comprehensive Health Insurance Plan

CHN: Child Neurology

Chng: change

CHO: carbohydrate

chol: cholesterol

chol est: cholesterol esters

CHP: Child Psychiatry

chpx: chickenpox

CHR: cercarien hüllen reaction

Chr: *Chromobacterium*

chr: chronic

c hr: candle hour

ChrBrSyn: chronic brain syndrome

Chron: chronological

CHSS: Cooperative Health Statistics System

CI:
cardiac index
chemotherapeutic index
clonus index
coefficient of intelligence
colour index
contamination index
coronary insufficiency
crystalline insulin

Ci: curie

CIB: International Council for Building Research Studies and Documentation

cib: *cibus* (L) food

CIBHA: congenital inclusion body haemolytic anaemia

CIC: cardio-inhibitor centre

CICU: Coronary Intensive Care Unit

CID:
chick infective dose
cytomegalic inclusion disease

CIEP: counterimmuno-electrophoresis

CIF: cloning inhibiting factor

CIFC: Council for the Investigation of Fertility Control

CIH:
carbohydrate-induced hyperglyceridaemia
Certificate in Industrial Health

CIM: cortically induced movement

CIOMS: Council for International

Organizations of Medical Sciences

cir: circular

circ:
circuit
circular
circulatory (tion)
circumcision(ed)

CIRM: Centro Internazionale Radio-Medico

CIS:
central inhibitory state
Chemical Information System

cit: citrate

cito disp: *cito dispensetur* (L) dispense quickly

CJD: Creutzfeldt–Jakob disease

CK:
creatine kinase
cyanogen chloride, a war gas

ck: check(ed)

CL:
chest and left arm lead (cardiology)
cholesterol-lecithin (test)
corpus luteum
critical list

CLA: cervicolinguoaxial

Cl:
chloride
chlorine (chemical symbol for)
clavicle
clinic
Clostridium (bacteriology)
closure

cl: centilitre, a hundredth part of a litre

ClAc: chloroacetyl

classif: classification

cldy: cloudy

Clin: clinical

clini: clinitest

Clin path: clinical pathology

Clin proc: clinical procedures

CLIP: corticotrophin-like intermediate lobe peptide

CLL:
cholesterol-lowering lipid
chronic lymphocytic leukaemia

Cl liq: clear liquid

CLML: Current List of Medical Literature

CLO: cod liver oil

Clon: *Clonorchis*
CIP: Clinical Pathology
cl.pal: cleft palate
CLR: chloride test (dentistry)
CLT: clot lysis time
CM:
  California mastitis (test)
  carboxymethyl
  Chick-Martin (coefficient)
  Chirurgiae Magister (L) Master
    in Surgery
  circular muscle
  congenital malformation
  copulatory mechanism
  contrast media
C&M: cocaine and morphine
  mixed
C$_m$:
  maximum clearance, with refer-
    ence to urea clearance, test
  curium (chemical symbol for)
cm:
  centimetre
  costal margin
  cras mane (L) tomorrow morn-
    ing
cm^3: cubic centimetre
CMA: Canadian Medical Association
CMB:
  carbolic methylene blue
  Central Midwives' Board
  chloromercuribenzoate
CMC:
  carboxymethyl cellulose
  carpometacarpal
CMD: count median diameter (of
  particles)
CME: continuing medical education
CMF: chondromyxoid fibroma
CMG: chopped meat glucose
  (agar)
CMH: congenital malformation of
  heart
CMHC: Community Mental Health
  Center
CMI:
  carbohydrate metabolism index
  cell-mediated immunity
  Commonwealth Mycological
    Institute
  Cornell Medical Index

CMIT: Current Medical Infor-
  mation and Terminology
CML: chronic myelocytic
  leukaemia
cmm: cubic millimetre
CMN: cystic medial necrosis (of
  aorta)
CMO: cardiac minute output
CMP: cytidine monophosphate
CMR: cerebral metabolic rate
CMRG: cerebral metabolic rate of
  glucose
cms: *cras mane sumendus* (L) to
  be taken tomorrow morning
cm/s: centimetres per second
CMSS: circulation, motor ability
  sensation, and swelling
CMT:
  California mastitis test
  Current Medical Terminology
CMV: cytomegalovirus
CN:
  caudate nucleus
  Charge Nurse
  chloroacetophenone, a war gas
  clinical nursing
  cranial nerve
  cyanogen radical
cn: *cras nocte* (L) tomorrow
  night
CNA: Canadian Nurses' Association
CNE: chronic nervous exhaustion
CNM: Certified Nurse-Midwife
CNR: Civil Nursing Reserve
CNS:
  central nervous system
  sulphocyanate
cns: *cras nocte sumendus* (L) to
  be taken tomorrow night
CO:
  carbon monoxide (chemical
    formula)
  cardiac output
  castor oil
  casualty officer
  centric occlusion
  crossover(s) (genetics)
C/O:
  check out
  complains of
CO$_2$: carbon dioxide (chemical
  formula)

Co:
  cobalt (chemical symbol for)
  coenzyme
^{60}**Co:** radioactive cobalt
co: *compositus* (L) a compound,
  compounded
CO I: coenzyme I, diphosphopyridine nucleotide (DPN)
CO II: coenzyme II, triphosphopyridine nucleotide (TPN)
CoA: coenzyme A
COAD: chronic obstructive airway
  disease
coag: coagulate(ion)
coag time: coagulation time
COBT: chronic obstruction of bili-
  ary tract
COC:
  cathodal opening contraction
  coccygeal
  combination (type) oral contraceptive
coch, cochleat: *cochlear,*
  cochleare, cochleatum (L) a
  spoonful, by spoonfuls
coch amp: *cochleare amplum* (L)
  tablespoon
coch mag: *cochleare magnum* (L)
  a large spoonful (about 14 ml)
coch med: *cochleare medium* (L)
  a dessert spoonful (about 7
  ml)
coch parv: *cochleare parvum* (L)
  a teaspoonful (about 4 ml)
COCl: cathodal opening clonus
coct: *coctio* (L) boiling
COD:
  cause of death
  chemical oxygen demand
  Council of Deans
cod: codeine
coeff: coefficient
COEPS: cortically originating
  extrapyramidal system
COGTT: cortisone (primed) oral
  glucose tolerance test
COH: carbohydrate
COHb: carboxyhaemoglobin
Col: cortisol
col:
  cola (L) strain
  colony (bacteriology)
  coloured

  column
colat: *colatus* (L) strained
COLD: chronic obstructive lung
  disease
colen: *colentur* (L) let them be
  strained
colet: *coleatur* (L) let it be strained
coll:
  collect(ion)
  college
  colloidal
  collyrium (L) an eyewash
collun: *collunarium* (L) nose wash
collut: *collutorium* (L) a mouth-
  wash
coll vol: collective volume
collyr: *collyrium* (L) an eyewash
COM: College of Osteopathic
  Medicine
commun dis: communicable disease
comp:
  compare
  compensated
  complaint
  composition
  compositus (L) compounded of
  compound
Comp case: Compensation
  (*workman's*) case
compd: compound
compl:
  completed
  complications
Complic: complications
compn: composition
COMT: catechol-*O*-methyl transferase
con: *contra* (L) against
conc: concentration(ed)
concd: concentrated
concentr: concentrated
concis: *concisus* (L) cut
concn: concentration(ate)
cond:
  condensed
  condition(s)
  conductivity
cond ref: conditioned reflex
cond resp: conditioned response
conf:
  confectio (L) a confection
  conference

cong: *congius* (L) gallon
congen: congenital
conj: conjunctiva
Cons: consultant(ing)
cons:
  conserva (L) keep, save
  consonans (L) tinkling
consperg: *consperge* (L) dust, sprinkle
const: constant
constit:
  constituent
  constitution(al)
cont:
  containing
  contents
  continue
  contra (L) against
  contusus (L) bruised
contag: contagious
conter: *contere* (L) rub together
contg: containing
contin: *continuetur* (L) let it be continued
contra: contraindicated
contralat: contralateral
cont rem: *continuantur remedia* (L) let the medicine be continued
contrit: *contritus* (L) broken, ground
contus: *contusus* (L) bruised
conv: convalescent
conv strab: convergent strabismus
COOH: carboxyl group (characteristic of organic acids)
coord: coordination
COP:
  change of plaster
  colloidal osmotic pressure
COPD: chronic obstructive pulmonary disease
COPE: chronic obstructive pulmonary emphysema
COPRO: coproporphyrin
COQ: ubiquinone
coq: *coque* (L) to boil
coq in sa: *coque in sufficiente aqua* (L) boil in sufficient water
coq sa: *coque secundum artem* (L) boil properly

coq simul (L) boil together
COR: cortisone
CoR: Congo red
cor: corrected(ion)
CORD: Commissioned Officer Residency Deferment (Program)
cort: cortex, cortical
COS:
  Canadian Ophthalmological Society
  Clinical Orthopedic Society
COSPAR: Committee on Space Research
COSTEP: Commissioned Officer Student Training and Extern Program
COTA: Certified Occupational Therapy Assistant
COTe: cathodal opening tetanus
COV: cross-over value (genetics)
CP:
  candle power
  capillary pressure
  cerebral palsy
  Certified Prosthetist
  chemically pure
  Child Psychiatry
  Child Psychology
  chloroquine-primaquine
  cleft palate
  cochlear potential
  code of practice
  combining power
  compensated base
  compound
  compressed (tablet)
  constant pressure
  coproporphyrin
  cor pulmonale (right ventricular failure)
  creatine phosphate (phosphocreatine)
C/P: cholesterol–phospholipid ratio
C&P:
  compensation and pension
  cystoscopy and pyelogram
Cp: chickenpox
cp:
  compare
  centipoise

CPA: chlorophenylalanine

C$_{PAH}$: *p*-aminohippuric acid clearance

CPAP: continuous positive airway pressure

CPB:
cardiopulmonary bypass
cetyl pyridinium bromide
competitive protein-binding

CPC:
Cerebral Palsy Clinic
chronic passive congestion
Clinical Pathological Conference

CPD:
citrate phosphate dextrose
contact potential difference
contagious pustular dermatitis
cyclopentadiene

CPE:
chronic pulmonary emphysema
corona penetrating enzyme
cytopathogenic effects

CPH: Certificate in Public Health

CPH 5: Cutter protein hydrolysate, 5% in water

CPI:
California Psychological Inventory
constitutional psychopathia inferior

CPIB: chlorophenoxyisobutyrate

cpl: complete

CPLM: cysteine-peptone-liver infusion (media)

CPK: creatine phosphokinase

CPM: counts per minute

CPP:
cerebral perfusion pressure
cyclopenteno-phenanthrene

CPPV: continuous positive pressure ventilation

CPR:
cardiac pulmonary reserve
cardiopulmonary resuscitation
centripetal rub
chlorophenyl red

CPRD: Committee on Prosthetics Research and Development

CPS: constitutional psychopathic state

cps: cycles (double vibrations) per second

CPT:
combining power test
Current Procedural Terminology

CPU: central processing unit (of computer)

CPZ: chlorpromazine

CQ:
chloroquine-quinine
conceptual quotient

CQM: chloroquine mustard

CR:
cardiorespiratory
centric relation
chest and right arm (lead)
clot retraction
coefficient of fat retention
colon resection
complete remission
conditioned reflex or response
cresyl red, an indicator
critical ratio
crown-rump (with reference to length of fetus)

Cr:
chromium (chemical symbol for)
cranial
creatinine
crown

^{51}Cr: radioactive sodium chromate

cr: *cras* (L) tomorrow

Cr&Br: crown and bridge

crast: *crastinus* (L) for tomorrow

CRBBB: complete right bundle branch block

CRD:
chronic renal disease
chronic respiratory disease
complete reaction of degeneration

CRE: cumulative radiation effect

crep: *crepitus* (L) crepitation

CRF:
chronic renal failure
coagulase reacting factor
corticotrophin-release factor

CRH: corticotrophin (ACTH)-releasing hormone

CRI:
chemical rust-inhibiting (germicide)
cold running intelligibility (with reference to test for hearing continuous speech)

CRL: Certified Record Librarian
CRM: cross-reacting material
Cr nn: cranial nerves
CRO:
  cathode ray oscilloscope
  centric relation occlusion
CROS: contralateral routing of signal
CRP: C-reactive protein
CrP: creatine phosphate
CRPA: C-reactive protein anti-serum
CRS:
  Chinese restaurant syndrome
  colon and rectal surgery
CRT:
  cardiac resuscitation team
  cathode ray tube
  complex reaction timer
CRTT: Certified Respiratory Therapy Technician
CRU: Clinical Research Unit
CRVS: California Relative Value Studies
crys: crystalline(ized)
cryst: crystalline(ized)
CS:
  Caesarean section
  Central Supply
  cerebrospinal
  chest strap
  chondroitin sulphate
  Christian Scientist
  Church of Scotland
  concentrated strength (of solutions)
  colla sinistra (L) with the left hand
  conditioned stimulus
  congenital syphilis
  conscious(ness)
  convalescent status
  coronary sclerosis
  corticosteroid
  current strength
  cycloserine
C&S: culture and sensitivity
Cs:
  caesium (chemical symbol for)
  case(s)
  conscious, consciousness
  standard clearance (with reference to urea clearance test)

cS: centistoke
CSA: chondroitin sulphate A
csc: *coup sur coup* (L) in small doses at short intervals
CSD: conditionally streptomycin dependent
CSF:
  cerebrospinal fluid
  colony stimulating factor
CSF-WR: cerebrospinal fluid-Wassermann reaction
CSM: cerebrospinal meningitis
CSMMG: Chartered Society of Massage and Medical Gymnastics
CSOM: chronic suppurative otitis media
CSP:
  Chartered Society of Physiotherapists
  Cooperative Statistical Program (for IUD data)
CSR:
  Cheyne-Stokes respiration
  corrected sedimentation rate
  cortical secretion rate (of adrenal)
CSS:
  chewing, sucking, swallowing
  subclinical scurvy syndrome
CSSD: Central Sterile Supply Department
CST: convulsive shock therapy
CSTI: Clearinghouse for Scientific and Technical Information
CSU:
  catheter specimen of urine
  Central Statistical Unit (of VDRL, q.v.)
CT:
  calcitonin
  carpal tunnel
  Cellular Therapy
  cerebral thrombosis
  clotting (coagulation) time
  coated tablet
  compressed tablet
  connective tissue
  continue treatment
  continuous-flow tub
  corneal transplant
  coronary thrombosis
  corrective therapist(y)

cystine-tellurite (medium)
cytotechnologist
Ct: *Ctenocephalides* (a genus of fleas)
CTA:
Canadian Tuberculosis Association
cyano-trimetay-androsterone
cyproterone acetate
CTa: catamenia (menstruation)
CTAB:
cetrimide
cetyltrimethyl-ammonium bromide
CTAC: Cancer Treatment Advisory Committee (HEW)
CTC: chlortetracycline
CTD: carpal tunnel decompression
CTP: cytidine triphosphate
CTR: cardiothoracic ratio
ctr: centre
CTS:
carpal tunnel syndrome
computerized topographic scanner
CTT: compressed tablet triturate
CTU: centigrade thermal unit
CT zone: chemoreceptor trigger zone (vomiting area in medulla)
CU:
clinical unit
Convalescent Unit
Cu: copper (chemical symbol for)
⁶¹Cu, ⁶⁴Cu: radioactive copper
cu: cubic
CuB: copper band (dentistry)
CUC: chronic ulcerative colitis
cu cm: cubic centimetre
CUG: cystourethrogram
cuj: *cujus* (L) of which, of any
cuj lib: *cujus libet* (L) of whatever you please
cult: culture (bacteriology)
cu mm: cubic millimetre
cur:
curative
current
curat: *curatio* (L) a dressing
CuSCN: cuprous thiocyanate
CV:
cardiovascular

cell volume
cerebrovascular
coefficient of variation
colour vision
concentrated volume (solutions)
conjugata vera (L) true conjugate diameter of pelvic inlet
conversational voice
corpuscular volume
cras vespere (L) tomorrow evening
cresyl violet
Cv: specific heat at constant volume
CVA: cerebrovascular accident
cva: costovertebral angle
CVD:
cardiovascular disease
color vision deviate
C-viruses: Coxsackie viruses
CVO:
Chief Veterinary Officer
conjugata vera obstetrica (L) obstetric conjugate diameter
CVP:
cell volume profile
central venous pressure
CVR:
cardiovascular renal (disease)
cardiovascular-respiratory
cerebrovascular resistance
CVS:
cardiovascular surgery
cardiovascular system
clean voided specimen
CVTR: charcoal viral transport medium
CW:
case work
chemical warfare
chest wall
Children's Ward
clockwise
continuous wave
crutch walking
CWBTS: capillary whole blood true sugar
CWI: cardiac work index
CWOP: childbirth without pain
CWS: cold-water soluble
cwt: hundredweight
CX:
cervix

chest X-ray
Cx: convex
Cy:
  cyanogen
  cyclonium (chemical symbol for)
cyath: *cyathus* (L) a glass
cyath vin: *cyathus vinarius* (L) a
  wineglass
cyc:
  cyclazocine
  cyclotron
CYL: casein yeast lactate (media)
cyl:
  cylinder
  cylindrical lens
CYS: cystoscopy
Cys: cysteine
Cys-cys: cystine
cytol: cytology(ical)
cyt sys:
  cytochrome system
CZI: crystalline zinc insulin

D

D:
  Symbol for vitamin D potency of
    good cod-liver oil
  da (L) give
  date
  daughter
  dead air space
  deciduous
  degree
  dermatologist(gy)
  detur (L) let it be given
  deuterium (heavy hydrogen)
  developed (SEE *w/d*)
  deviation
  diagnosis
  diameter
  difference
  diffusing capacity
  diffusion constant
  dioptry
  disease
  District Administrator
  divorced
  dog (veterinary medicine)
  donor
  Doriden (glutethimide)

  dosis (L) dose
  drive or drive state
  duodenum
  dwarf
d:
  deci (prefix)
  density
  dexter (right)
  dextrorotatory
  died (deceased)
  dies (L) day
  dioptre
  distal
  dorsal
  dose
  doubtful
  duration
δ**:** delta (fourth letter of Greek
  alphabet)
D-:
  dextrorotatory
  A chemical prefix (small capital)
    which designates that a sub-
    stance has the configuration
    of glyceraldehyde
  In carbohydrate nomeclature,
    the symbol designates the
    configuration of the *highest
    numbered* asymmetric car-
    bon atom (EX *D-glucose*)
  In amino acid nomenclature, the
    symbol designates the con-
    figuration to which the *lowest
    numbered* asymmetric car-
    bon atom belongs (EX *D-
    threonine*)
d-: Chemical abbreviation for *dex-
    tro*, to the right or clockwise,
    especially with reference to
    direction in which a plane of
    polarized light is rotated
D_1**,** D_2**, etc:** first dorsal (thoracic)
    vertebra, second dorsal ver-
    tebra, etc
17-D: a modified yellow fever
    virus
D 40: uroselectan (Iopax) (a com-
    pound used in radiography)
D 860: Orinase (an oral hypo-
    glycaemic sulphonamide)
D_0**:** diffusing capacity of oxygen
DA:
  degenerative arthritis

delayed action (with reference to drugs)
Dental Assistant
developmental age
diphenylchlorarsine (a war gas)
Diploma in Anaesthetics
disability assistance
D/A: discharge and advise
da:
daughter
day
deca (prefix)
DAB: 4-dimethylamino-azobenzene
DAB 6: benzinum petrolii
D and C: dilatation and curretage
DAD: dispense as directed
DADAVS: Deputy Assistant Director Army Veterinary Services
DADDS: diacetyl diamino-diphenylsulphone
DADMS: Deputy Assistant Director of Medical Services (Armed Forces)
DADS: Director Army Dental Service
DAH: disordered action of the heart
DALA: delta-aminolaevulinic acid
DAM:
degraded amyloid
diacetylmonoxime
Dictionary of Abbreviations in Medicine
dam: decameter
DAO: duly authorised officer
DAP:
diaminopimelic acid
dihydroxyacetone phosphate
direct latex agglutination pregnancy (test)
draw a person test
DAPT: amiphenasole; 2: 4-diamino-5-phenylthiazole
DAS: dextroamphetamine sulphate
DAT:
delayed action tablet
diet as tolerated
differential agglutination titre
differential aptitude test
dau: daughter

DAV&RS: Director Army Veterinary and Remount Services
DB:
Baudelocque's diameter (external conjugate diameter of pelvis)
distobuccal
dry bulb
Db: dubhium (ytterbium) (chemical symbol for)
db: decibel
DBA: dibenzanthracene
DBC: dye-binding capacity
DBE: A synthetic oestrogen
DBI:
development at birth index
phenformin (an oral hypoglycaemic agent)
phenethyguanide
DBM: diabetic management
DBO: distobucco-occlusal
DBP:
diastolic blood pressure
dibutylphthalate
distobuccopulpal
DBS:
despeciated bovine serum
Division of Biological Standards
DBT: dry bulb temperature
DBW: desirable body weight
DC:
Dental Corps
diagnostic centre
diphenylcyanoarsine (a war gas)
direct current
discharged
discontinue
distocervical
Doctor of Chiropractic
donor's cells (corpuscles)
D/C: discontinue
D&C:
dilatation and curettage
Drugs and Cosmetics
DCA:
desoxycholate citrate agar
deoxycorticosterone acetate (SEE *DOCA*)
DCC: Day Care Center
DCc: double concave
DCF: direct centrifugal flotation

DCG: deoxycorticosterone glucoside

DCH: Diploma in Child Health

DCh: *Doctor Chirurgiae* (L) Doctor of Surgery

DCHN: dicyclohexylamine nitrite

DCI:
dichloroisoprenaline
dichloroisoproterenol

DCLS: deoxycholate citrate lactose saccharose (agar)

DCN: delayed conditioned necrosis

DCOG: Diploma of College of Obstetricians and Gynecologists

DCP:
dicalcium phosphate
Diploma in Clinical Pathology
District Community Physician

DCR: direct cortical response

DCT: distal convoluted tubule (of kidney)

DCTMA: deoxycorticosterone-trimethyl-acetate

DCU: dichloral urea

DCVO: Deputy Chief Veterinary Officer

DCx: double convex

DD:
dependent drainage
developmental disability
differential diagnosis
disc diameter
double diffusion (test)
dry dressing

dd: *detur ad* (L) let it be given to

DDA:
An acetic derivative of DDT excreted in urine
Dangerous Drugs Act

DDC: diethyldithiocarbamine

DDD:
dehydroxydinapthyl disulphide
dichloro-diphenyl-dichloro-ethane (an insecticide, SYN: *TDE*)

DDE: A derivative of DDT stored in fat

DDIB: Disease Detection Information Bureau

dd in d: *de die in diem* (L) from day to day

DDM: Diploma in Dermatological Medicine

DDMS: Deputy Director of Medical Services (Armed Forces)

DDO: Diploma in Dental Orthopaedics

DDR: Diploma in Diagnostic Radiology

DDS:
dapsone (diphenyl sulphone)
diamino diphenyl sulphone
Doctor of Dental Surgery

DDSc: Doctor of Dental Science

DDSO: diamino-diphenyl-sulphoxide

DDST: Denver Developmental Screening Test

DDT: dichloro-diphenyl-trichloroethane (an insecticide)

DDVP: 2 2-dichlorvinyldimethyl phosphate (Dichlorvos)

DE: digestive energy

D&E: dilatation and evacuation

DEA:
dehydroepiandrosterone
Drug Enforcement Administration

DEAE: diethylaminoethanol

dearg pil: *deargentur pilulae* (L) let the pills be silverized

deaur pil: *deaurentur pilulae* (L) let the pills be gilded

DEB: diethylbutanediol

deb spis: *debita spissitudine* (L) of the proper consistency

dec:
decanta (L) pour off
decompose
decrease

decd: deceased, dead

decomp: decompose

decompn: decomposition

decoct: *decoctum* (L) decoction

decr: decreased or diminished

dec (R): decrease, relative

decub: *decubitus* (L) lying down

DED: delayed erythema dose

de d in d: *de die in diem* (L) from day to day

DEF: Dental formula designating: number of teeth for filling; e, number for extraction; f, number of filled teeth (with reference to deciduous teeth)

def:
defaecation
deficient
define(ition)

defib: defibrillate

defic:
deficiency
deficit

deform: deformity

deg:
degeneration
degree

degen: degeneration

deglut: *deglutiatur* (L) let it be swallowed

DEHS: Division of Emergency Health Services

dej: dento-enamel junction

Del: delivery

del: delusion

deliq: deliquescent

Dem: Demerol (meperidine hydrochloride)

denat: denatured

Dent:
dental
dentistry
dentition

dent: *dentur* (L) give, let it be given

dent tal dos: *dentur tales doses* (L) give of such doses

DEP: diethylpropanediol

Dep: dependents

dep: *deputatus* (L) purified

DEPA: diethylene phosphoramide

depr: depressed

DeR: reaction of degeneration (SEE *RD*)

deriv: derivative of or derived from

Derm: dermatology

DES:
diethylstilboestrol
Doctor's Emergency Service

desat: desaturated

desc: descendent(ing)

dest: *destilla* (L) distil and *distillatus* (L) distilled

destil: *destilla* (L) distil

DET: diethyltryptamine

det: *detur* (L) let it be given

determin: determination

det in dup: *detur in duplo* (L) let twice as much be given

det in 2 plo: *detur in duplo* (L) let twice as much be given

detn: detention

d et s: *detur et signatur* (L) let it be given and labelled

DEV: duck egg (embryo) virus

dev: deviation

devel: development

DF:
decapacitation factor (with reference to sperm)
degree of freedom (of movement)
dorsiflexion

DFC: dry-filled capsules

DFDT: difluoro-diphenyl-trichloro-ethane (an insecticide)

DFO: District Finance Officer

DFP: diisopropyl fluorophosphate

DG:
diglyceride
distogingival

dg: decigram (a tenth part of a gram)

DGMS: Director General of Medical Services (Armed Forces)

DGO: Diploma in Gynaecology & Obstetrics

DH:
Day Hospital
dehydrocholic acid
dehydrogenase
delayed hypersensitivity

DHA: dehydroepiandrosterone

DHAS: dehydroepiandrosterone sulphate

DHE 45: dihydroergotamine

DHEW: Department of Health, Education, and Welfare (US)

DHg: Doctor of Hygiene

DHIA: dehydroisoandrosterol

DHIC: dihydroisocodeine

DHMA: dehydroxymandelic acid

DHO: deuterium hydrogen (protium) oxide

DHO 180: dihydroergocornine

DHPG: dehydroxyphenylglycol

DHR: delayed hypersensitivity reactions

D-5-HS: dextrose (5%) in Hartman's solution
DHSM: dihydrostreptomycin
DHSS: Department of Health and Social Security (UK)
DHT:
dihydrotachysterol
dihydrotestosterone
dihydrothymine
DHyg: Doctor of Hygiene
DI:
deterioration index
diabetes insipidus
distoincisal
double indemnity
Di: didymium (chemical symbol for)
dia: diathermy
diab: diabetic
DIAC: diiodothyroacetic acid
diag:
diagnosis, diagnostic
diagonal
diagram
diam: diameter
dias: diastolic
diath: diathermy
DIB: butyl 3:5-di-iodo-4-hydroxybenzoate
DIC: disseminated intravascular coagulopathy or coagulation
dick: ethyldichloroarsine (a war gas)
dict: dictionary
dieb alt: *diebus alternus* (L) on alternate days
dieb tert: *diebus tertius* (L) every third day
diff:
difference
differential blood count
diff diag: differential diagnosis
DIFP: diisopropyl fluorophosphonate
Dig: *digeratur* (L) it be digested
DIH: Diploma in Industrial Health
DIHPPA: diiodohydroxyphenylpyruvic acid
dil: *dilue, dilutus* (L) dilute, diluted
dilat: dilatation(ed)
dild: diluted
diln: dilution
diluc: *diluculo* (L) at daybreak

dilut: *dilutus* (L) dilute
dim:
dimidius (L) one-half
diminutus (L) diminished
d in p aeq: *divide in partes aequales* (L) divide into equal parts
DIP: distal interphalangeal (joint)
DipAmerBdP&N: Diplomate American Board of Psychiatry and Neurology
DipBact: Diploma in Bacteriology
diph: diphtheria
diph-tet: diphtheria-tetanus
diph-tox: diphtheria toxoid (plain)
diph-tox AP: diphtheria toxoid (alum precipitated)
DipMicrobiol: Diploma in Microbiology
Dir: director
dir: *directione* (L) directions
dir prop: *directione propria* (L) with the proper directions
direct prop: *directione propria* (L) with the proper directions
dis:
disabled
disease
distance
disc: dicontinue
disch: discharge(ed)
disloc: dislocation
disod: disodium
disp:
dispensa (L) dispense
dispensary
dissd: dissolved
dissem: disseminated
dist:
distance
distilla (L) distil
dist f: distinguished from
distn: distillation
DIT: diiodotyrosine
div:
divide (L) divide
division
divid: divide
div in par aeq: *dividatur in partes aequales* (L) divide into equal parts
DJD: degenerative joint disease
dkg: decagram

dkm: decameter
DL:
 danger list
 difference limen (threshold)
 distolingual
 Donath-Landsteiner (test)
dl: decilitre (one tenth of a litre)
DLa: distolabial
DLaI: distolabioincisal
DLaP: distolabiopulpal
DLE: disseminated lupus ery-
 thematosus
DLF: Disabled Living Foundation
DLI: distolinguoincisal
DLLI: dulcitol lysine lactose iron
 (agar)
DLO: Diploma in Laryngol & Otol
DLP: distolinguopulpal
DM:
 diabetes mellitus
 diastolic murmur
 diphenylaminearsine chloride
 (Adamsite) (a war gas)
 Doctor Medicinae (L) Doctor of
 Medicine
dm: decimetre (one tenth of a
 metre)
DMA: dimethylamine
DMAC: dimethylacetamide
DMBA: dimethylbenzanthracene
DMC:
 dimethylcarbinol (an insecticide)
 dimite (1, 1-bis-[p-chloro-
 phenyl] ethanol) (an acari-
 cide)
DMCTC: dimethylchlor-
 tetracycline
DMD: Doctor of Dental Medicine
DMDT: dimethoxydiphenyl tri-
 chloroethane; methoxychlor
 (Marlate) (an insecticide)
DME: Director of Medical Edu-
 cation
DMF: In dentistry, formula rep-
 resenting number of decayed,
 missing, and filled teeth (with
 reference to permanent teeth)
DMHS: Director Medical & Health
 Services
DMP: dimethylphthalate (an insect
 repellent)
DMPA: Depo-medroxypro-
 gesterone acetate

DMPE: dimethoxyphenyl-
 ethylamine
DMR: Diploma in Medical Radiol-
 ogy
DMRD: Diploma in Medical
 Radio-Diagnosis
DMRE: Diploma in Medical
 Radiology and Electrology
DMRT: Diploma in Medical
 Radio-Therapy
DMS:
 dermatomyositis
 Director of Medical Services
 (Armed Forces)
 Doctor of Medical Science
DMSO: dimethylsulphoxide
DMSS: Director of Medical &
 Sanitary Services
DMT: dimethyltryptamine
DMV: Doctor of Veterinary
 Medicine
DN:
 dibucaine number
 dicrotic notch
 Diploma in Nursing
 District Nurse
D/N: dextrose–nitrogen (ratio)
Dn: dekanem
dn: decinem (one tenth of a nem,
 q.v.)
DNA:
 deoxyribonucleic acid
 did not attend
DNase: desoxyribonuclease
DNB:
 dinitrobenzene
 Diplomate of the National Board
 of Medical Examiners
DNBP: dinitrobutylphenol
DNC: did not come
DNCB: dinitrochlorobenzene
DNE: Director of Nursing Edu-
 cation
DNFB: dinitrofluorobenzene
DNO: District Nursing Officer
DNOC: Dinitro-ortho-cresol
DNP:
 2-4-dinitrophenyl group
 do not publish
DNPM: dinitrophenyl-morphine
DNS: Dinoyl sebacate
DNTP: diethyl-nitrophenyl thio-
 phosphate (an insecticide)

DO:
- diamine oxidase
- Diploma in Ophthalmology
- dissolved oxygen
- disto-occlusal
- Doctor of Optometry
- Doctor of Osteopathy
- doctor's orders

do:
- *dictum* (L) the same, as before
- ditto

DOA: dead on arrival

DOAC: Dubois oleic albumin complex (bacteriology)

DOB:
- date of birth
- doctor's order book

DObstRCOG: Diploma of the Royal College of Obstetricians & Gynaecologists

DOC: desoxycorticosterone

doc: document

DOCA: desoxycorticosterone acetate

DOCG: deoxycorticosterone glucoside

DOD: Department of Defense

DOE:
- desoxyephedrine hydrochloride
- dyspnoea on exertion

DOM: SEE *STP*

dom: domestic

DOMS: Diploma in Ophthalmic Medicine & Surgery

DON: diazooxo-L-norleucine

don: *donec* (L) until

donec alv sol fuerit: *donec alvus soluta fuerit* (L) until the bowels are opened

DOPA: 3:4-dihydroxyphenylalanine

DOPAMINE: dihydroxyphenylethylamine

dopase: dopa oxidase

DOph: Doctor of Ophthalmology

dorna: desoxyribose nucleic acid (SEE *DNA*)

dos:
- dosage
- *dosis* (L) dose

DOSC: Dubois oleic serum complex (bacteriology)

DOSS: distal over-shoulder strap

DP:
- deep pulse
- dementia precox
- diffusion pressure
- digestible protein
- diphosgene (a war gas)
- diphosphate
- diproprionate
- *directione propria* (L) with proper direction
- displaced person
- distopulpal
- Doctor of Pharmacy
- donor's plasma

DPA:
- diphenylamine
- dipicolinic acid

DPD:
- Department of Public Dispensary
- diphenamid
- Diploma in Public Dentistry

DPDA: phosphorodiamidic anhydride

DPF: Dental Practitioners' Formulary

DPG: diphosphoglycerate

DPH:
- Department of Public Health
- diphenylhydantoin
- Diploma in Public Health
- Doctor of Public Health

DPh: Doctor of Philosophy

DPhysMed: Diploma in Physical Medicine

DPM:
- Diploma in Psychological Medicine
- discontinue previous medication
- Doctor of Podiatric Medicine

DPN: diphosphopyridine nucleotide

DPNH: disphosphopyridine nucleotide (reduced form)

DPPD: diphenyl-*p*-phenylenediamine

DPT:
- diphosphothiamine
- diphtheria, pertussis, tetanus
- dipropyltryptamine

DQ: deterioration quotient

DR:
- Delivery Room

diabetic retinopathy
diagnostic radiology
Diploma in Radiology
dorsal root (of spinal nerve)
reaction of degeneration (with reference to muscle fibres)
Dr: Doctor
dr:
dorsal root (of spinal nerves)
drachm (dram)
dressing
dr ap: drachm apothecaries' weight
DRF: daily replacement factor (of lymphocytes)
dRib: deoxyribose
DRNA: desoxyribose nucleic acid (SEE *DNA*)
DRnt: diagnostic roentgenology
DRO: Disablement Resettlement Officer
DRP: *Deutsches Reichs-Patent* (German patent)
DrPH: Doctor of Public Health
DRQ: discomfort relief quotient
drsg: dressing
DRVO: Deputy Regional Veterinary Officer
DS:
dead-air space
density (optical) standard
dilute strength (of solutions)
dioptric strength
Doctor of Science
donor's serum
double-stranded (DNA)
double strength
Down's syndrome
D/S:
dextrose and saline
dominance and submission
D-5-S: dextrose (5%) in saline
DSC:
disodium cromoglycate
Doctor of Surgical Chiropody
DSc: Doctor of Science
DSCS: disodium cromoglycate
DSD: dry sterile dressing
DSS: dioctyl sodium sulpho-succinate (Aerosol OT, a wetting agent)
DSSc: Diploma in Sanitary Science

DST:
daylight saving time
desensitization test
dexamethasone suppression test
dihydrostreptomycin
DSUH: direct suggestion under hypnosis
DT:
delirium tremens
diphtheria-tetanus
dispensing tablet
distance test
duration of tetany
D/T: deaths: total ratio
DTCD: Diploma in Tuberculosis & Chest Diseases
dtd: *datur talis dosis* (L) give of such a dose
dtdNo iv: *dentur tales doses No. iv* (L) let four such doses be given
DTH: Diploma in Tropical Hygiene
DTM: Diploma in Tropical Medicine
DTMA: desoxycorticosterone trimethylacelate
DTM&H: Diplomate of Tropical Medicine and Hygiene
DTN: diphtheria toxin, normal
DTNB: dithionitrobenzene
DTP:
diphtheria, tetanus, pertussis
distal tingling on percussion
DTR: deep tendon reflex
DTT: diphtheria-tetanus toxoid
DTVM: Diploma in Tropical Veterinary Medicine
DU:
diagnosis undetermined
density (optical) unknown
dog unit (with reference to adrenal cortical hormones)
duodenal ulcer
dulc: *dulcis* (L) sweet
duod: duodenum
dup: duplicate
dur: *duris* (L) hard
dur dolor: *durante dolore* (L) while the pain lasts
DV:
dependant variable
dilute volume (of solutions)

distemper virus
domiciliary visit
dv: double vibrations
D&V: diarrhoea and vomiting
DVA: duration of voluntary
apnoea(test)
DVH: Diploma in Veterinary
Hygiene
DVM: Doctor of Veterinary
Medicine
DVMS: Doctor of Veterinary
Medicine and Surgery
DVR: Department of Vocational
Rehabilitation
DVS:
Doctor of Veterinary Science
Doctor of Veterinary Surgery
DVSc: Doctor of Veterinary
Science
DVSM: Diploma of Veterinary
State Medicine
DVT: deep venous thrombosis
DW: distilled water
D/W: dextrose in water
D-5-W: dextrose (5%) in water
dwt: pennyweight
Dx: diagnosis
DXM: dexamethasone (test for
adrenocortical function)
DXR: deep X-ray
DXRT: deep X-ray therapy
Dy: dysprosium (chemical symbol
for)
dyn: dyne
DZ: dizygotic

E

E:
electrode potential
electromotive force
emmetropia
energy
enzyme
Escherichia (bacteriology)
ester
experimenter
expired gas
eye
e:
electric charge

electron
ex (L) from
ε: epsilon (fifth letter of Greek
alphabet)
E_0: electric affinity
E3: lachesine chloride
4E: four plus oedema
EA:
educational age
erythrocyte antibody
estimoautumal (malaria)
ea: each
EAA: essential amino acid
EAC:
erythrocyte antibody
complement
external auditory canal
EACA: e-aminocaproic acid
EACD: eczematous allergic
contact dermatitis
ead: *eadem* (L) the same
EAE: experimental allergic
encephalomyelitis
EAHF: eczema, asthma, and hay
fever
EAM: external acoustic meatus
EAP: epiallopregnanolone (an
androgen in pregnancy
urine)
EaR: *Entartungs-Reaktion* (Ger)
reaction of degeneration (SEE
RD)
EB:
elementary body
Epstein-Barr (virus)
EBF: erythroblastosis fetalis
EBI: emetine bismuth iodide
EBM: expressed breast milk
EBS:
electric brain stimulator
Emergency Bed Service
EBV: Epstein-Barr virus
EC:
electron capture
enteric coated (with reference to
tablets)
entering cmplaint
Enzyme Commission
expiratory centre
extracellular
E/C: oestrogen to creatinine (ratio)
E-C mixture: ether-chloroform
mixture

ECBO: enteric cytopathogenic bovine orphan (virus)

ECC: electrocorticogram

ECDO:
enteric cytopathic dog orphan (virus)

ECF:
Extended Care Facility
extracellular fluid

ECFMG: Educational Commission for Foreign Medical Graduates

ECFMS: Educational Council for Foreign Medical Students

ECG: electrocardiogram(-graph)

ECHO:
echoencephalogram (sonoencephalon)
enterocytopathogenic human orphan (virus)

ECI: extracorporeal irradiation

Eclec: eclectic

ECMO: enteric cytopathic monkey orphan (virus)

E coli: *Escherichia coli*

ECP:
estradiol cyclopentane-oproprionate
free cytoporphyrin in erythrocytes

ECPO: enteric cytopathogenic porcine orphan (virus)

ECPOG: electrochemical potential gradient

ECS: electroconvulsive shock

ECSO: enteric cytopathic swine orphan (virus)

ECT:
electroconvulsive (electro-shock) therapy
enteric coated tablet

ECV: extracellular volume

ED:
effective dose
Entner-Doudoroff (metabolic pathway)
epidural
erythema dose
ethyl dichlorarsine (a war gas)

Ed: editor

ed: edition

ED$_{50}$: median effective dose

EDB: early dry breakfast

EDC: expected date of confinement

EDD:
enzyme-digested delta (endotoxin)
expected date of delivery

edent: edentulous

E-diol: estradiol

EDN: electrodesiccation

EDP:
electronic data processing
end diastolic pressure

EDR:
effective direct radiation
electrodermal response

EDTA: ethylenediaminetetra-acetic acid (edathamil) (a chelating agent)

EDV: end diastolic volume

EDx: electrodiagnosis

EE:
embryo extract
equine encephalitis
eye and ear

E-E: erythematous-edematous(reaction)

EEC: European Economic Community

EE3ME: ethinyloestradiol 3-methyl ether

EEE: eastern equine encephalitis

EEG: electroencephalograph (-gram)

EENT: eyes, ears nose, and throat

EES: ethyl ethanesulphate

EF:
edema factor
equivalent focus
extrinsic factor

EFA: essential fatty acids

EFE: endocardial fibro-elastosis

EFF: efficiency

eff:
effects
efferent

effect: effective

effer: efferent

EFP: effective filtration pressure

EFR: effective filtration rate

eg: *exempli gratia* (L) for example

EGF: epidermal growth factor

EGTA: ethylene glycol tetra-acetic acid

EH: enlarged heart
E&H: environment and heredity (psychology)
eH: oxidation-reduction potential
EHBF: extrahepatic blood flow
EHC:
  enterohepatic circulation
  enterohepatic clearance
EHD: epizootic haemorrhagic disease (of poultry)
EHL: effective half-life (of radioactive substances)
EHP:
  di-(2 ethylhexyl) hydrogen phosphate
  extra high potency
EHPT: Eddy hot plate test
EHSDS: Experimental Health Service Delivery System
EIRv: extra incidence rate in vaccinated groups
EIRnv: extra incidence rate in non-vaccinated groups
EIS: Epidemiological Investigational Service
EIT: erythroid iron turnover
EJ: elbow jerk
EJP: excitatory junction potential
ejusd: *ejusdem* (L) of the same
EKG:
  electrocardiograph(-gram) (SEE *ECG*)
  epidemic keratoconjunctivitis
EKY: electrokymograph (-gram)
EL:
  early latent
  exercise limit
ELB: early light breakfast
elec:
  electric(al)
  electricity
elect: *electuarium* (L) electuary
elem: elementary
elev: elevator(ion) (ate)
elix: *elixir* (L) elixir
EM: electron microscope(scopy)
E-M: Embden-Meyerhof (glycolytic pathway)
e/m: ratio of charge to mass (of an electron)
E&M: endocrine and metabolism
Em: emmetropia (normal vision)
Emb: embryology

EMB: eosin-methylene blue (agar)
embryol: embryology
EMC: encephalomyocarditis
EMCRO: Experimental Medical Care Review Organization
emend: *emendatis* (L) emended
emer: emergency
EMF:
  electromotive force
  endomyocardial fibrosis
  erythrocyte maturation factor
EMG:
  electromyograph(-gram)
  exomphalos, macroglossia, and giantism (syndrome)
EMIC: emergency maternity and infant care
EMO: Epstein and Macintosh, Oxford (ether inhaler and Oxford bellow)
emot: emotion(al)
emp:
  emplastrum (L) a plaster
  ex modo prescripto (L) after the manner prescribed, as directed
emp vesic: *emplastrum vesicatorium* (L) a blistering plaster
EMS:
  early morning specimen
  Emergency Medical Service
  ethyl methane sulphonate
emu: electromagnetic unit
emuls: *emulsio* (L) an emulsion
EN: erythema nodosum
en:
  enema
  ethylene diamine (in chemical formulas)
ENA: extractable nuclear antigens
END: Enhancement Newcastle Disease
Endo: endodontics
Endocrin: endocrinology
enem: enema
ENG: etectronystagmograph (-gram)
Eng: England
ENP: ethyl-*p*-nitrophenylthio-benzene-phosphate
ENR: extrathyroidal neck radio-activity

ENT: ears, nose, and throat
Entom: entomology
environ: environment(al)
EOA: examination, opinion, and advice
E of M: error of measurement
EOG: electro-oculogram
EOM:
  extraocular movement
  extraocular muscles
Eos: eosinophil(s)
Eosins: eosinophils
EOU: epidemic observation unit
EP:
  ectopic pregnancy
  electrophoresis
  endogenous pyrogen
  endpoint
  extreme pressure
  protoporphyrin (free in erythrocytes)
EPA:
  erect posterior-anterior
  Environmental Protection Agency (US)
EPC: epilepsy partialis continua
Ep cells: epithelial cells
EPEC: enteropathogenic *Escherichia coli*
EPF: exophthalmos-producing factor
EPG: eggs per gram (parasitology)
epid: epidemic
Epil: epilepsy (tic)
epineph: epinephrine
epis: episiotomy
epistom: *epistomium* (L) a stopper
epith:
  epithelial cells
  epithelium(-al)
EPP: end-plate potential
EPPS: Edwards Personal Preference Schedule
EPR: electrophrenic respiration
EPS: exophthalmos-producing substance (of anterior pituitary)
ep's: epithelial cells
EPSP: excitatory post-synaptic potential
EPTS: existed prior to service

EQ: educational quotient
eq:
  equation
  equivalent
equip: equipment
equiv: equivalent
ER:
  emergency room
  endoplasmic reticulum
  environmental resistance
  equivalent roentgen (unit)
  evoked response
  extended release
  external resistance
Er:
  erbium (chemical symbol for)
  erythrocyte
ERA: Electroshock Research Association
ERBF: effective renal blood flow
ERC: ECHO-rhino-coryza (viruses)
ERD: evoked response detector
ERDA: Energy Research and Development Administration
ERF: Education and Research Foundation (AMA)
ERG: electroretinogram
ERIA: electroradio-immuno assay
ERP: effective refractory period
ERPF: effective renal plasma flow
ERV: expiratory reserve volume
ERY: erysipelas
Ery: *Erysipelothrix*
ES:
  elastic suspensor
  electrical stimulus
  Emergerncy Service
  enema saponis
  enzyme substrate
Es: einsteinium (chemical symbol for)
ESA: Entomological Society of America
ESB: eletrical stimulation to brain
Esch: *Escherichia*
ESCN: electrolyte and steroid-produced cardiopathy characterized by necrosis
ESE: *electrostatische Einheit* (Ger) electrostatic unit

ESF: erythropoietic stimulating factor (SEE *EMF*)
ESN: educationally subnormal
esoph: esophagus
ESP:
  end systolic pressure
  extrasensory perception
esp: especial(ly)
espec: especial(ly)
ESR:
  electron spin resonance
  erythrocyte sedimentation rate
EST: electroshock therapy
est: estimated
esth: esthetic
est wt: estimated weight
esu: electrostatic unit
E substance: excitor substance
ET:
  educational therapy
  endotracheal tube
ET-3: erythrocyte triiodothyronine (also T-e)
Et: ethyl (chemical symbol for)
et al:
  et alibi (L) and elsewhere
  et alii (L) and others
etc: *et cetera* (L) and others of the like kind, and so forth
ETF: electron-transferring flavo-protein
eth: ether
ETIO: etiocholandone
etiol: etiology
EtOH: ethyl alcohol
ETP: electron transport particle
et seq: *et sequentes* (L) and those that follow
ETT: exercise tolerance test
ETU:
  Emergency and Trauma Unit
  Emergency Treatment Unit
EU:
  Entropy Unit
  Enzyme Unit
Eu: europium (chemical symbol for)
EUA: examination under anaesthetic
EUROTOX: European Committee on Chronic Toxicity Hazards
EUV: extreme ultraviolet laser

EV:
  evoked response
  extravascular
ev:
  electron volt
  eversion
EVA:
  ethyl violet azide (broth)
  ethylene vinyl acetate
evac: evacuated
eval: evaluate (ation)
evap: evaporated
ever: eversion
EW: Emergency Ward
EWL: evaporative water loss
ex:
  exaggerated
  examined
  example
  exercise
ex aff: *ex affinis* (L) of affinity
exag: exaggerated
exam: examination
exc: except(ed)
exer: exercise
ex gr: *ex grupa* (L) of the group of
exhib: *exhibeatur* (L) let it be given
exp:
  expecting(ed)
  experiment(al)
  expired
expect: *expectorant* (L) expectorant
exper: experiment(al)
expir: expiration(atory)
expt:
  expected
  experimental
exptl: experimental
EXREM: external radiation dose
Ext: extraction (dentistry)
ext:
  extend (L) spread
  extensor(ion)
  external
  extractum (L) extract
  extremity
extd: extracted
ext fl: fluid extract
ext rot: external rotation
Ez: eczema

F

F:
  facies
  Fahrenheit (temperature
    scale)
  failure
  family
  farad (unit of electrical
    capacity)
  fasting (test)
  father
  Fellow
  female
  fetal
  fertility
  fibrous (with reference to
    proteins)
  field of vision
  fine
  finger
  flow (of blood)
  fluorine (chemical symbol for)
  focal length
  foil (dentistry)
  formula(ary)
  fractional (with reference to frac-
    tional composition of gases)
  free
  French (catheter size)
  frontal
  full (with reference to diet)
  function

f:
  fac, fiat, fiant (L) make, let it be
    made, let them be made
  farad (unit of electrical capacity)
  fluid
  focal
  forma (L) form
  frequency
  from

F_1: first filial generation

F_2:
  second filial generation
  zinc oxide-eugenol cement
    (dentistry)

f-12: freon (a refrigerant)

FA:
  fatty acid
  febrile antigens
  field ambulance
  filterable agent
  first aid
  fluorescent antibody
  folic acid
  fortified aqueous (with reference
    to solutions)
  Freund's adjuvant
  functional activities

FAA sol: formalin, acetic, alcohol
  solution (a fixative)

FAB:
  antigen-binding fragments
  functional arm brace

FACA: Fellow of the American
  College of Anaesthetists

FACC: Fellow of the American
  College of Cardiologists

FACD: Fellow of the American
  College of Dentists

FACFS: Fellow of the American
  College of Foot Surgeons

FACOG: Fellow of the American
  College of Obstetricians and
  Gynecologists

FACP: Fellow of the American
  College of Physicians

FACR: Fellow of the American
  College of Radiologists

FACS: Fellow of the American
  College of Surgeons

FACSM: Fellow of the American
  College of Sports Medicine

FACT: Flanagan Aptitude
  Classification Test

FAD: flavine adenine dinucleotide

$FADH_2$: flavine adenine
  dinucleotide, reduced form

FADN: flavine adenine
  dinucleotide

Fahr: Fahrenheit

Fam: family

FAMA: Fellow of the American
  Medical Association

Fam per par: familial periodic
  paralysis

Fam phys: family physician

FANS: Fellow of the American
  Neurological Society

FANY: First Aid Nursing
  Yeomanry

FAPA:
  Fellow of the American
    Psychiatric Association
  Fellow of the American
    Psychoanalytical Association
F&R: force and rhythm (of pulse)
FAO: Food and Agricultural
  Organization (of the United
  Nations)
FAPHA: Fellow of the American
  Public Health Association
FAR: flight aptitude rating
far: faradic
FAS: Federation of American
  Scientists
fasc: *fasciculus* (L) bundle
FASEB: Federation of American
  Societies for Experimental
  Biology
FB:
  finger breadth
  foreign body
FBA: Fellow of the British
  Academy
FBCOD: foreign body cornea right
  eye
FBCOS: foreign body cornea left
  eye
FBI: flossing, brushing and
  irrigation (dentistry)
FBN: Federal Bureau of Narcotics
FBPsS: Fellow of the British
  Psychological Society
FBS:
  fasting blood sugar
  feedback signal
  feedback system
  fetal bovine serum
Fc: crystallizable fragment (of Ig)
fc: foot candle
FCAP: Fellow of the College of
  American Pathologists
FCC: Federal Communications
  Commission
FCCP: Fellow of the American
  College of Chest Physicians
FCGP: Fellow of the College of
  General Practitioners
FChS: Fellow of the Society of
  Chiropodists
fcly: face lying
FCP: final common pathway
  (neurology)

FCPS: Fellow of the College of
  Physicians and Surgeons
FCPSA: Fellow of the College of
  Physicians and Surgeons of
  S Africa
FCRA: Fellow of the College of
  Radiologists of Austra-
  lasia
FCS:
  Fellow of the Chemical Society
  fetal calf serum
FCT: food composition table
FD:
  fan douche
  fatal dose
  focal distance
  forceps delivery
  freeze-dried
FD$_{50}$: median fatal dose (that
  fatal to 50% of test
  subjects)
FDA:
  Food and Drug Administration
  frontodextra-anterior (L) right
  fronto-anterior (position of
  fetus)
FD&C: Food, Drug, and Cosmetic
  (Act)
FDD: Food and Drugs Directorate
  (Canada)
FDDC: ferric dimethyl dithio-
  carbonate (a fungicide)
FDF: fast death factor
fdg: feeding
FDI: Federation Dentaire Internationale
FDIU: fetal death in utero
FDNB: fluorodinitrobenzene
FDO: Fleet Dental Officer
FDP:
  fibrin degradation product
  frontodextra posterior (L)
  right front-posterior position of
  fetus)
  fructose diphosphate
FDS: Fellow in Dental Surgery
FDSRCSEng: Fellow in Dental
  Surgery of the Royal College
  of Surgeons of England
FDT: *frontodextra transversa* (L)
  right fronto-transverse position of fetus)
FE: fetal erythroblastosis

Fe: ferrum (L) (chemical symbol for iron)

^{59}Fe: radioactive iron

feb dur: *febre durante* (L) while the fever lasts

FEBS: Federation of European Biochemical Societies

FECG: fetal electrocardiogram

FECT: fibro-elastic connective tissue

Fed:
federal
federation

Fed spec: federal specifications

FEHBP: Federal Employees Health Benefits Program

FEKG: fetal electrocardiogram

Fel: Fellow

FEM: *femoris* (L) thigh

fem:
female
feminine

Fem intern: *femoribus internus* (L) at the inner side of the thighs

fertd: fertilized

ferv: *fervens* (L) boiling

FEV$_1$: forced expiratory volume in one second

FF:
fat free
filtration fraction
fixing fluid
foster father
fresh frozen

ff:
following
force fluid

FFA:
Fellow of the Faculty of Anaesthetists
free fatty acid

FFARCS: Fellow of the Faculty of Anaesthetists, RCS

FFC: free from chlorine

FFD: focus film distance (X-ray)

FFDRCS: Fellow of the Faculty of Dental Surgery Royal College of Surgeons

FFDW: fat-free dry weight

FFHom: Fellow of the Faculty of Homoeopathy

FFI: free from infection

FFP: fresh frozen plasma

FFR: Fellow of the Faculty of Radiologists

FFS: fat-free supper

FFT: flicker fusion threshold

FFWW: fat-free wet weight

FH:
family history
fetal heart
Frankfort horizontal (plane of skull)

fh: *fiat haustus* (L) let a draught be made

FHIP: Family Health Insurance Plan

FHNH: fetal heart not heard

FHR: fetal heart rate

FHS: fetal heart sounds

FHT: fetal heart tone

FI: fixed internal (reinforcement)

FIAT: Field Information Agency, Technical (U.S. Reports)

fibrill: fibrillation

FIC: Fellow of the Institute of Chemistry

FICA: Federal Insurance Contribution Act (Social Security)

FICD: Fellow of the International College of Dentists

FICS: Fellow of the International College of Surgeons

FID: flame ionization detector

FIFRA: Federal Insecticide, Fungicide and Rodenticide Act

fig:
figuratively
figure

FIGLU: formiminoglutamic acid

FIH: fat-induced hyperglycaemia

fil: filamentous

filt *filtra* (l) filter

FIMLT: Fellow of the Institute of Medical Laboratory Technology

FIN: fine intestinal needle

FInstSP: Fellow of the Institute of Sewage Purification

F-insulin: fibrous insulin

fist: fistula

F-J: Fisher-John (melting point method)

FJRM: full joint range of movement
Fl: focal length
fL: foot Lambert
fl:
  flexion
  fluidium (L) fluid
FLA: *frontolaeva anterior* (L) fronto-anterior (position of fetus)
fla: *fiat lege artis* (L) let it be done according to rule
flac: flaccid
flav: *flavus* (L) yellow
fld: fluid
fl dr: fluid drachm (dram)
fldxt: *fluidextractum* (L) fluid extract
FLEX: Federal Licensing Examination
flex: flexor(ion)
FLK: funny looking kid (paediatrics)
flocc: flocculation
flor: *flores* (L) flowers
fl oz: fluid ounce
FLP: *frontolaeva posterior* (L) left frontoposterior (position of fetus)
FLS:
  Fellow of the Linnaean Society
  fibrous long spacing (collagen)
FLT: *frontolaeva transversa* (L) left frontotransverse (position of fetus)
fluor: fluoroscopy(escent)
fluores: fluorescent
FM:
  flavin mononucleotide
  formerly married
  foster mother
  frequency modulation
  fusobacteria micro-organisms
Fm: fermium (chemical symbol for)
fm: *fiat mistura* (L) make a mixture
FMC: Foundation for Medical Care
FMD: foot and mouth disease
FME: full mouth extraction
FMF:
  familial Mediterranean fever
  fetal movement felt
FMG: Foreign Medical Graduates

FMN: flavin mononucleotide
FMP:
  Family Nurse Practitioner
  first menstrual period
FMS:
  fat-mobilizing substance
  full mouth series
FMX: full mouth radiography (dentistry)
F-N: finger to nose
Fneg: false negative
f-number: focal length (of a lens)
FO:
  foramen ovale
  fronto-occipital
FOB:
  faecal occult blood
  feet out of bed
fol:
  folium (L) a leaf
  following
FOR: forensic (pathology)
for: foreign
form:
  formation
  formula
fort: *fortis* (L) strong
Found: foundation
FP:
  Family Planning
  family practice
  Family Practitioner
  flat plate
  flavin phosphate (riboflavin-5'-phosphate)
  flavoprotein
  frozen plasma
fp:
  fiat potio (L) let a potion be made
  foot-pound
  forearm pronated
  freezing point
FPA: Family Planning Association
FPC:
  Family Planning Clinic
  Family Practitioner Committee
  fish protein concentrate
FPH₂: flavin phosphate, reduced
f pil: *fiant pilulae* (L) let pills be made
f pil xi: *fac pilulas xi* (L) make 11 pills
fpm: feet per minute

FPM test: filter paper microscopic test

FPS: Fellow of the Pharmaceutical Society

fps:
feet per second
foot-pound-second

F&R: force and rhythm (of pulse)

FR:
failure rate (with reference to contraception)
fixed ratio
flocculation reaction

Fr:
francium (chemical symbol)
French

fr: from

FRACP: Fellow of the Royal Australian College of Physicians

FRACS: Fellow of the Royal Australasian College of Surgeons

Fract:
fraction
fracture

fract dos: *fracta dosi* (L) in divided doses

FRAI: Fellow of the Royal Anthropological Institute

FRC:
Federal Radiation Council
frozen red cells
functional residual capacity (of lungs)

FRCGP: Fellow of the Royal College of General Practitioners

FRCOG: Fellow of the Royal College of Obstetricians and Gynaecologists

FRCP: Fellow of the Royal College of Physicians

FRCPath: Fellow of the Royal College of Pathologists

FRCP(C): Fellow of the Royal College of Physicians of Canada

FRCPE: Fellow of the Royal College of Physicians of Edinburgh

FRCP(Glasg): Fellow of the Royal College of Physicians and Surgeons of Glasgow *qua* Physician

FRCPI: Fellow of the Royal College of Physicians of Ireland

FRCS: Fellow of the Royal College of Surgeons

FRCS(C): Fellow of the Royal College of Surgeons of Canada

FRCSE: Fellow of the Royal College of Surgeons of Edinburgh

FRCS(Glasg): Fellow of the Royal College of Physicians and Surgeons of Glasgow *qua* Surgeon

FRCSI: Fellow of the Royal College of Surgeons in Ireland

FRCVS: Fellow of the Royal College of Veterinary Surgeons

frem: *fremitus vocalis* (L) vocal fremitus

freq: frequency

FRES: Fellow of the Royal Entomological Society

FRF: follicle-stimulating hormone releasing factor

FRFPSG: Fellow of the Royal Faculty of Physicians and Surgeons of Glasgow

FRH: follicle-stimulating hormone-releasing hormone

FRIC: Fellow of the Royal Institute of Chemistry

frict: friction

Fried test: Friedman test (for pregnancy)

frig: *frigidus* (L) cold

FRIPHH: Fellow of the Royal Institute of Public Health & Hygiene

FRJM: full range joint movement

FRMS: Fellow of the Royal Microscopical Society

FROM: full range of movement

FRS:
Fellow of the Royal Society
ferredoxin-reducing substance

FRSA: Fellow of the Royal Society of Arts

FRSE: Fellow of the Royal Society of Edinburgh

FRSH: Fellow of the Royal Society of Health

FRSPS: Fellow of the Royal Society of Physicians and Surgeons (Glasgow)

FRT: full recovery time

fru: fructose

fruat: *frustrillatum* (L) in small pieces

FS:
   factor of safety
   forearm supinated
   frozen section
   full and soft (diet)

FSA: Federal Security Administration

fsa: *fiat secundum artem* (L) let it be done skilfully

fsar: *fiat secundum artem reglas* (L) let it be made according to the rules of the art

FSC: Food Standards Committee (of Ministry of Agriculture, Fisheries, and Food) (UK)

FSD: focus skin distance (X-ray)

FSF: fibrin stabilizing factor (XIII)

FSH: follicle-stimulating hormone

FSHRF: follicle-stimulating hormone releasing factor

FSHRH: follicle-stimulating hormone releasing hormone

FSM: flying spot microscope

FSMB: Federation of State Medical Boards (US)

FSR: Fellow of the Society of Radiographers

FSR-3: isoniazid

FSU: Family Service Unit

FT:
   follow through (after Ba. meal)
   formol toxoid
   free thyroxine
   full term

ft:
   fac, fiat, fiant (L) make, let it be made, let them be made
   foot or feet

FTA: fluorescent treponemal antibody (test)

FTA-ABS: fluorescent treponemal antibody-absorption (test)

FTBD:
   fit to be detained
   full term born dead

FTC: Federal Trade Commission

ft c: foot candle

ft cataplasm: *fiat cataplasma* (L) let a poultice be made

ft cerat: *fiat ceratum* (L) let a cerate be made

ft chart vi: *fiant chartulae vi* (L) let six powders be made

ft collyr: *fiat collyrium* (L) let an eyewash be made

ft emuls: *fiat emulsio* (L) let an emulsion be made

ft enem: *fiat enema* (L) let an injection (for rectum) be made

ft garg: *fiat gargarisma* (L) let a gargle be made

FTI: free thyroxine index

ft infus: *fiat infusum* (L) let an injection be made (for urethra)

ftL: foot Lambert

ft lb: foot pound

ft linim: *fiat linimentum* (L) let a liniment be made

FTM: fractional test meal

ft mas: *fiat massa* (L) let a mass be made

ft mass div in pil xiv: *fiat massa et divide in pilulae xiv* (L) let 14 pills be made

ft mist: *fiat mistura* (L) let a mixture be made

FTND: full term normal delivery

ft pil xxiv: *fiat pilulae xxiv* (L) let 24 pills be made

ft pulv: *fiat pulvis* (L) let a powder be made

ft solut: *fiat solutio* (L) let a solution be made

ft suppos: *fiat suppositorium* (L) let a suppository be made

ft ung: *fiat unguentum* (L) let an ointment be made

FTT: failure to thrive

FU:
   faecal urobilinogen
   fluorouracil
   follow up
   fractional urinalysis

Fu: Finsen unit (for ultraviolet rays)

FUB: functional uterine bleeding

FUDR: floxuridine
FUM: fumarate
funct: function(al)
FUO: fever of undetermined origin
FVC: forced vital capacity
f vs: *fiat venaesectio* (L) let the patient be bled
FW: forced whisper
fw: fresh water
FWA: Family Welfare Association
FWPCA: Federal Water Pollution Control Administration
Fx: fracture
FY: full year
FZS: Fellow of the Zoological Society

G

G:
  gap (in cell cycle)
  gas
  gastrin
  gauge
  gauss (in magnetism)
  giga (prefix)
  gingival
  globular (with reference to proteins)
  globulin
  glucose
  goat (in veterinary medicine)
  gold inlay (dentistry)
  gonidial (with reference to colonies of bacteria)
  gram(s)
  gravitation constant (Newtonian constant)
  Greek
  green (an indicator colour)
  guanine
  guanosine
  A unit of force of acceleration (in aviation medicine)

g:
  acceleration due to gravity
  gender
  gram(s)
  group

γ:
  gamma (third letter of Greek alphabet)
  immunoglobulin
γ**G:** immunoglobulin G
GI, GII, GIII: number of previous pregnancies
G_4: dichlorophen (dihydroxy-dichlorodiphenyl urethane)
G-6-P: glucose-6-phosphate
G_{11}: hexachlorophene
GA:
  gastric analysis
  general anesthesia
  gingivoaxial
  glucuronic acid
  guessed average
  gut-associated
Ga: gallium (chemical symbol for)
ga: gauge (of needles)
GABA: gamma-aminobutyric acid
gal:
  galactose
  gallon
GALT: gut-associated lymphoid tissue
galv: galvanic
gang: ganglion
gangl: ganglion(ic)
garg: *gargarismus*(L) gargle
GARP: Global Atmospheric Research Program
GAS:
  general adaptation syndrome
  generalized arteriosclerosis
  gastroenterology
Gastroc: gastrocnemius (muscle)
GB:
  gall bladder
  goofball (barbiturate pill)
  Guillain-Barré (syndrome)
GBA: gingivobuccoaxial
GBH: gamma benzene hydrochloride (an isomer of BHC)
GBM: glomerular basement membrane
GBS:
  gall bladder series
  glycerine buffered saline
GC:
  ganglion cells
  gas chromotography

glucocorticoid
gonococcal infection (gonorrhoea)
gonococcus(al)
guanine-cystosine

g-cal: gram calorie (small calorie)

GCFT:
gonorrhoea complement fixation test

GC type: guanine, cytosine type (with reference to pentose nucleic acids)

GCWM: General Conference on Weights and Measures

Gd: gadolinium (chemical symbol for)

GDH: growth and differentiation hormone (in insects)

GDMO: General Duties Medical Officer

GDP: guanosine diphosphate

GE: gastroenterology (itis)

Ge: germanium (chemical symbol for)

g-e: gravity eliminated

GEF: gonadotrophin enhancing factor

gel: gelatin(ous)

gel quav: *gelatina quavis* (L) in any kind of jelly

gen:
general
genus (L) genus

genet: genetics

gen et sp nov: *genus et species nova* (L) new genus and species

genit: genitalia

gen'l: general

gen nov: *genus novum* (L) new genus

gen proc: general procedure

Ger:
geriatrics
German

Geriat: geriatrics

Gerontol: gerontology(ist)

GET: gastric emptying time

GF:
germ-free
glass factor (tissue culture)
glomerular filtrate
growth fraction

G-F: globular-fibrous (with reference to proteins)

gf: gram-force

G-forces: acceleration forces

GFR: glomerular filtration rate

GG:
gammaglobulin
glycylglycine

GGE: generalized glandular enlargement

GGG: *gummi guttae gambiae* (L) gamboge

GH:
General Hospital
growth (somatotrophic) hormone (of anterior pituitary)

G+H: Gibb & Helmholtz (equation)

GHAA: Group Health Association of America

GHRF: growth hormone releasing factor

GHRH: growth hormone releasing hormone

GHRIH: growth hormone release-inhibiting hormone

GI:
gastrointestinal
globin insulin
growth-inhibiting

GHRIH: growth hormone release-inhibiting factor

GIH: gastrointestinal hormone

GII: gastrointestinal infection

ging: *gingiva* (L) gum

g-ion: gram-ion

GIP: gastric inhibitory polypeptide

GIS: gastrointestinal series

GIT: gastrointestinal tract

GIX: DFDT, *q.v.*

Gk: Greek

GL: greatest length (with reference to embryos)

GL54 athomin

Gl: glucinium (chemical symbol for) (SEE *Be*)

gl: gill

g/l: grams per litre

GLA: gingivolinguoaxial

glac: glacial

gland:
glandula (L) a gland
glandular

GLC: gas-liquid chromatography
glc: glaucoma
GLI: glucagon-like immuno-
    reactivity
Gln: glutamine
Glob:
    globular
    globulin
Glu:
    glutamic acid
    glutamin
GLX: An insecticide
Gly: glycine
glyc:
    glycerin
    glyceritum (L) glycerite
GM:
    General Medicine
    grand mal
    monosialoganglioside
gm: gram(s)
g/m: gallons per minute
GMC:
    General Medical Council
    grivet monkey cell (line)
GMK: green monkey kidney (cells)
gm/l: grams per litre
gm-m: gram-metre
g-mol: gram-molecule
GMP: guanosine monophosphate
GMS: General Medical Services
GM&S: general medicine and
    surgery
GMT: Greenwich Mean Time
GMW: gram molecular weight
GN:
    glomerular nephritis
    Graduate Nurse
    Gram-negative
G/N: glucose: nitrogen (ratio in
    urine examination)
Gn: gonadotrophin
GNC:
    general nursing care
    General Nursing Council
GnRH: gonadotrophin-releasing
    hormone
G&O: gas and oxygen
GOE: gas, oxygen, ether (in
    anaesthesia)
GOK: God only knows
Gold sol: colloidal gold curve
GOR: general operating room

GOT: glutamic oxalo-acetic trans-
    aminase
Gov: governmental
GP:
    general paralysis
    general paresis
    general practitioner
    geometric progression
    Gram-positive
    group
    guinea pig
GPB: glossopharyngeal breathing
GPD: glucose-6-phosphate de-
    hydrogenase
G-6PD: glucose-6-
    phosphate-dehydrogenase
GPI: general paresis of the insane
Gply: gingivoplasty
GPM: general preventive
    medicine
GPRA: General Practice Reform
    Association
GPS: guinea pig serum
GPT: glutamic pyruvic trans-
    aminase
GpTh: group therapy
GPU: guinea-pig unit
GR:
    gamma ray
    gastric resection
    general research
    glutathione reductase
gr:
    gamma roentgen
    grain(s)
    gravity
grad:
    gradient
    graduate(d)
GRAE: generally regarded as
    effective
gran: *granulatus* (L) granulated
GRAS: generally regarded as safe
    (with reference to food addi-
    tives)
grav:
    gravid (pregnant)
    gravity
grd: ground
GRF: growth hormone-releasing
    factor
gros: *grossus* (L) coarse
grp: group

GS:
general surgery
glomerular sclerosis
g/s: gallons per second
GSA: general somatic afferent (nerve)
GSC: gravity settling culture (plate)
GSD: glycogen storage disease
GSE: general somatic efferent (nerve)
GSH: glutathione (reduced form)
GSR:
galvanic skin response
generalized Schartzman reaction
GSSG: glutathione (oxidized form)
GSW: gunshot wound
GT:
generation time
genetic therapy
glucose tolerance
group therapy
gt: *gutta* (L) drop
g/t:
granulation time
granulation tissue
GTF: glucose tolerance factor
GTH: gonadotrophic hormone
GTN: glomerulo-tubulo-nephritis
GTP: guanosine triphosphate
GTR: granulocyte turnover rate
GTT: glucose tolerance test
gtt: *guttae* (L) drops
GU:
gastric ulcer
genitourinary
glycogenic unit
gonococcal urethritis
gravitational ulcer
guid: guidance
gutt quibusd: *guttis quibusdam* (L) with a few drops
guttat: *guttatim* (L) drop by drop
GV: gentian violet
GVA: general visceral afferent (nerve)
GVE: general visceral efferent (nerve)
GVH: graft versus host (reaction)
Gvty: gingivectomy
GW: glycerine in water
GYN: gynaecology(ist)

H

H:
Symbol for Hauch, designating motile or flagellate type of micro-organism
flagella (with reference to antigens) (bacteriology)
heavy
henry (symbol for unit of electrical inductance)
heroin
Holzknecht unit
homosexual
hormone
horse (in veterinary medicine)
human
hydrogen (chemical symbol for)
hyoscine (scopolamine)
hypermetropia
hypodermic
mustard gas (a war gas)
Symbol for oersted, a unit of magnetizing force
h:
haustus (L) a draft
hecto (prefix)
height
henry (symbol for unit of electrical inductance)
hora (L) hour
horizontal
Planck's constant (symbol for)
quantum constant (symbol for)
H^+: hydrogen ion (symbol for)
^1H: protium (light hydrogen) (chemical symbol for)
H 1: para-aminobenzoic acid
^2H: deuterium (heavy hydrogen) (chemical symbol for)
H 2: diethylaminoethanol
H_3: procaine hydrochloride
^3H: deuterium (heavy hydrogen) (chemical symbol for)
HA:
haemadsorption (test)
haemagglutination
haemolytic anaemia
headache
hepatitis associated (virus)

Ha: absolute hypermetropia
HA1: haemadsorption (virus, type 1)
HAA:
  haemolytic anaemia antigen
  hepatitis associated antigen
H&A Ins: Health and Accident Insurance
habit: habitat
HAc: acetic acid
HAD: hospital administration(or)
haem: haemolysis (with reference to blood fragility test)
haemat:
  haematocrit
  haematology
haematol: haematology(ist)
haemorrh: haemorrhage
HAGG: hyperimmune antivariola gamma globulin
HAI: haemagglutination inhibition (procedure)
halluc: hallucination
H antigens: antigens localized in flagella of motile bacteria
HAS:
  highest asymptomatic (dose)
  hypertensive arteriosclerotic
H&ASHD: hypertension and arteriosclerotic heart disease
HASP: Hospital Admission and Surveillance Program
haust: *haustus* (L) a draft
HAV: hepatitis A virus
HB:
  heart block
  hepatitis B
Hb: haemoglobin
HbA: adult haemoglobin
HBAg: hepatitis B antigen
HB$_c$Ag: hepatitis B core antigen
HBD: hydroxybutyrate dehydrogenase
HBF: hepatic blood flow
HbF: fetal haemoglobin
HbO$_2$: oxy haemoglobin
HBP: high blood pressure
HbP: primitive (fetal) haemoglobin
HbS: sickle-cell haemoglobin
HB$_s$AG: hepatitis B surface antigen
HBSS: Hank's balanced salt solution

HBV: hepatitis B virus
HC:
  handicapped
  home care
  Hospital Corps
  house call
  hydrocarbon
  hydrocortisone
hc: *honoris causa* (degrees)
HCC: hepatitis contagiosa canis (virus)
HC3: Hemicholinium No. 3
HCD: homologous canine distemper antiserum
HCF: highest common factor
HCG: human chorionic gonadotrophin
HCH: hexachlorocyclohexane (benzene hexachloride; Lindane)
HcImp: hydrocolloid impression (dentistry)
HCR: hydrochloric acid (chemical formula for)
HCN: hydrocyanic acid (chemical formula for)
HCO$_3$: bicarbonate ion (chemical formula for)
H'crit: haematocrit
HCS:
  Hospital Car Service
  human chorionic somatomammotrophin (HPL)
HCT: human chorionic (placental) thyrotrophin
Hct: haematocrit
HCVD: hypertensive cardiovascular disease
HD:
  haemolysing dose
  Hansen's disease (leprosy)
  hearing distance
  heart disease
  herniated disc
  high density
  hip disarticulation
  Hodgkin's disease
hd: *hora decubitis* (L) at bedtime
HDA: hydroxy dopamine
HDC: histidine decarboxylase
HDD: Higher Dental Diploma
HDL: high density lipoprotein

HDLW: distance at which a watch is heard with left ear

HDN: haemolytic disease of the newborn

HDP: hexose diphosphate

HDRW: distance at which a watch is heard with right ear

HDU: haemodialysis unit

HE: human enteric

H&E:
haematoxylin and eosin
haemorrhage and exudate
heredity and environment

He: helium (chemical symbol for)

HEAT: human erythrocyte agglutination test

hebdom: *hebdomada* (L) a week

HED: *Haut-Einheits-Dosis* (Ger) unit skin dose (of roentgen rays)

HEENT: head, ears eyes, nose, throat

HEK: human embryonic kidney (cells)

HEL:
hen's egg-white lysozyme
human embryonic lung (cells)

HELA: Helen Lake (tumour cells)

HeLa cells: a continuous cell line used for tissue cultures

HEMAT: haematology

hemi:
hemiparalysis
hemiplegia

HEP:
high egg passage (strain of virus)
high energy phosphate

HEPA: high effieiency particulate air (filter)

herb recent: *herbarium recentium* (L) of fresh herbs

hered: heredity

hern: hernia, herniated

HETP: hexaethyltetraphosphate

HEW: Health, Education and Welfare (Dept of)

HF:
Hageman factor (in blood plasma)
hard filled (capsules)
hay fever
heart failure
high frequency

Hf: hafnium (chemical symbol)

hf: half

HFC: hard filled capsules

HFR: high frequency of recombination

Hfr: high frequency

HFT: high frequency transduction

HG: human gonadotrophin

Hg:
haemoglobin
hydrargyrum (L) mercury (chemical symbol for)

hg: hectogram (100 grams)

hgb: haemoglobin

HGA: homogentisate

HGF: hyperglycaemic-glyco-genolytic factor (glucagon)

Hg-F: fetal haemoglobin

HGG: human gamma globulin

HGH: human growth hormone

HGO: hepatic glucose output

HH:
hard of hearing
Henderson and Haggard (inhaler)
Home Help

HHb: reduced haemoglobin

HHD: hypertensive heart disease

HHHO: hypotonia-hypomentia-hypogonadism-obesity

HHT: hereditary haemorrhagic telangiectasia

H+Hm: compound hypermetropic astigmatism

HI:
haemagglutination inhibition
Hospital Insurance
hydriotic acid

Hi: histidine

HIAA: hydroxyindole-acetic acid

HIC: Heart Information Center

HID: headache, insomnia, depression (syndrome)

HIFC: hog intrinsic factor con-centrate

HIg: human immunoglobulin

H inf: hypodermoclysis infusion

Hint: Hinton (flocculation test for syphilis)

HIO:
hypoiodism
iodic acid

HIOMT: hydroxyindol-O-methyl transferase

HIP:
Health Insurance Plan
hydrostatic indifference point

His: histidine

Hist: history

Histol: histology

HIT: haemagglutination inhibition test (for pregnancy)

HJ: Howell-Jolly (bodies)

HJR: hepatojugular reflex (reflux)

HK cells: human kidney cells

H-K: hands to knee

HL:
half-life (of radioactive element)
Hygienic Laboratory (SEE *USHL*)
hypertrichosis lanuginosa

H/L: hydrophile/lipophile (number)

HI: latent hypermetropia, hyperopia

hl: hectolitre (100 litres)

H&L: heart and lungs

HLA: homologous leucocytic antibodies

HLB: hydrophile-lipophile balance (with reference to surfactants)

HLR: heart-lung resuscitation

HM: hand movements

Hm: manifest hypermetropia

hm: hectometre (100 metres)

HMB: homatropine methyl bromide

HMC:
heroin, morphine, cocaine
hydroxymethyl cystosine

HMD: hyaline membrane disease

HME:
heat, massage, exercise
hydroxymethyl glutaryl

HMG: human menopausal gonadotrophin

HMM:
heavy meromysin (of muscle)
hexamethylmelamine

HMMA: 4-hydroxy-3-methoxymandelic acid

HMO:
Health Maintenance Organization
heart minute output

HMP: hexose monophosphate

HMPA: hexamethylphosphoramide

HMT: human molar thyrotrophin

HMU: hydroxymethyl uracil

HMX: heat-massage-exercise

HN: Head Nurse

hn: *hoc nocte* (L) tonight

HNC: hypothalamic-neurohypophyseal complex

HNP: herniated nucleus pulposus

HNV: has not voided

HO: House Officer

H/O: history of

Ho: holmium (chemical symbol for)

HOCM: hypertrophic obstructive cardiomyopathy

hoc vesp: *hoc vespere* (L) this evening, tonight

HOD: hyperbaric oxygen drenching

HofF: height of fundus

Hoff: Hoffman (reflex)

Homeop: homeopathy

Homo: homosexual

Homolat: homolateral

HOP: high oxygen pressure

hor: horizontal

hor decu : *hora decubitus* (L) at bedtime

hor interm: *horis intermediis* (L) at the intermediate hours

hor som: *hora somni* (L) at bedtime

hor un spatio: *horae unius spatio* (L) at the end of one hour

HOS: human osteosarcoma

Hosp: hospital

Hosp Ins: hospital insurance

HOT: human old tuberculin

HP:
handicapped person
high potency
high power
high pressure
highly purified
hot pack or pad
House Physician
hydrostatic pressure
hyperphoria
hypertension + proteinuria

H&P: history and physical (examination)

Hp: haptoglobin
HPA: 4-ethylsulphonyl-naphthalene-1-sulphonamide
HPC: hydroxyphenyl-cinchoninic acid
H-PD: Hough-Powell digitizer
HPF: high-power field
HPG: human pituitary gonado-trophin
HPI: history of present illness
HPL:
  human parotid lysozyme
  human placental lactogen
HPN: hypertension
HPP:
  hydroxyphenyl pyruvate
  4-hydroxypyrazolo-pyrimidine
HPr: human prolactin
HPS: high protein supplement
HPT: human placenta thyrotrophin
HR:
  heart rate
  heterosexual relations (scale)
hr: hour
HRA: Health Resources Adminis-tration
HRE: high resolution electro-cardiography
HRL: head rotated left
HRP: horseradish peroxidase
HRR: head rotated right
HS:
  half strength
  Hartman's solution
  head sling
  heart sounds
  herpes simplex
  homologous serum
  horse serum
  hour of sleep
  House Supervisor
  House Surgeon
hs: *hora somni* (L) at bedtime
H&S: hysterotomy and steril-ization
HSA:
  Health Services Administration
  Hospital Savings Association
  human serum albumin
HS-CoA: coenzyme A, reduced
HSD: hydroxysteroid

  dehydrogenase
HSG: herpes simplex genitalis
HSL: herpes simplex labialis
HSMHA: Health Services and Mental Health Administration (HEW)
HSV: herpes simplex virus
H&T: hospitalization and treat-ment
HT:
  home treatment
  hydrotherapy
  hypermetropia (with L or R)
  hypodermic tablet
5-HT: 5-hydroxytryptamine (serotonin)
5-HTP: 5-hydroxytryptophan
HT: total hypermetropia
ht:
  heart tones
  height
  high tension
HTB: hot tub bath
HTC: hepatoma cells
HTF: heterothyrotrophic factors
HTH: homeostatic thymus hormone
HTST: high temperature-short time (pasteurization)
HU:
  Harvard University
  hyperaemia unit
HUS: haemolytic uremic syn-drome
HV: hyperventilation
HVA: homovanillic acíd
HVD: hypertensive vascular disease
HVG: host versus graft (response)
HVH: Herpes virus hominis
HVL: half value layer
HW: housewife
HWS: hot water soluble
HWY: hundred woman years (of exposure)
Hx:
  history
  hypoxanthine
Hy hypermetropia
hydr: hydraulic
hydrarg: *hydrargyrum* (L) mercury
Hydro: hydrotherapy

hydrox: hydroxyline
Hyg: hygiene
HYP: hypnosis
Hyp:
    hydroxyproline
    hyperresonance
    hypertrophy
Hypn: hypertension
hypno: hypnotism(sis)
Hypo: hypodermic injection
Hypox: hypophysectomized
Hypro: hydroxyproline
hys: hysteria(cal)
Hz: hertz (one cycle/sec)

I

I:
    incisor (permanent)
    index
    induction
    inhibitor
    intensity of magnetism
    internist
    iodine (chemical symbol for)
i:
    incisor (deciduous)
    insoluble
    optically inactive
^{125}I, ^{130}I, ^{131}I: radioactive iodine
IA:
    impedance angle
    intra-arterial
    intra-atrial
IAA:
    indole-3-acetic acid
    International Antituberculosis
        Association
IAB: Industrial Accident Board
IAEA: International Atomic Energy
    Agency
IAFI: infantile amaurotic familial
    idiocy
IAGP: International Association of
    Geographic Pathology
IAGUS: International Association
    of Genito-Urinary Surgeons
IAMM: International Association of
    Medical Museums
IAO:
    immediately after onset

intermittent aortic occlusion
IAPB: International Association for
    Prevention of Blindness
IAPP: International Association for
    Preventative Pediatrics
IAS: intra-amniotic saline
    (infusion)
IASD: interatrial septal defect
IAT: iodine azide test
IATA: International Air Transport
    Association
IB:
    immune body
    inclusion body
    index of body build
    infectious bronchitis
ib: *ibidem* (L) in the same place
IBC: iron-binding capacity
IBI: intermittent bladder irrigation
ibid: *ibidem* (L) in the same place;
    the same (authors)
IBP:
    International Biological Program
    iron-binding protein
IBR: infectious bovine rhino-
    tracheitis
IBT: isatin-beta-
    thiosemicarbasone
IBU: International Benzoate Unit
IBV: infectious bronchitis vaccine
IBW: ideal body weight
IC:
    inspiratory capacity
    inspiratory centre
    intensive care
    intercostal
    interstitial cells
    intracardiac
    intracellular
    intracerebral
    intracutaneous (injection)
ic: *inter cibos* (L) between meals
ICAA: Invalid Children's Aid
    Association
ICAV: intracavity
ICBP: intracellular binding
    proteins
ICC:
    Information Centre Complex
    Internal Conversion Coefficient
    (radiology)
ICCR: International Committee for
    Contraceptive Research

ICD:
  Institute for Crippled and Disabled
  intrauterine contraceptive device
ICDA: International Classification of Diseases, Adapted
ICDH: isocitric dehydrogenase
ICF
  indirect centrifugal flotation
  Intensive Care Facility
  Intermediate Care Facility
  intracellular fluid
ICG: indocyanine green
ICH: infectious canine hepatitis
ICLA: International Committee on Laboratory Animals
ICM: intercostal margin
ICN: International Council of Nurses
I, C, PM, M: incisors, canines, premolars, molars (When each is followed by a fraction, the entire expression is the formula of permanent dentition)
ICR: distance between iliac crests
ICRP: International Commission on Radiological Protection
ICRU: International Commission on Radiological Units and Measurements
ICS:
  impulse-conducting system
  Intensive Care, Surgical
  intercostal space
  International College of Surgeons
ICSH: interstitial cell-stimulating hormone (LH)
ICSU: International Council of Scientific Unions
ICT:
  icterus
  inflammation of connective tissue
  insulin coma therapy
ICU: Intensive Care Unit
ICUMSA: International Commission for Uniform Methods of Sugar Analysis
ID:
  inclusion disease

  index of discrimination
  infectious disease(s)
  infective dose
  inhibitory dose
  inside diameter
  intradermal(ly)
id: *idem* (L) the same
ID$_{50}$: median infective dose
I&D: incision and drainage
id ac: *idem ac* (L) the same as
idon vehic: *idoneo vehiculo* (L) in a suitable vehicle
IDP:
  immunodiffusion procedures
  inosine diphosphate
IDPN: B-iminodiproprionitrile
IDS: Investigative Dermatological Society
IDU: iododeoxyuridine (idoxuridine)
IDV: intermittent demand ventilation
IE:
  Immunitäts Einheit (Ger)
  immunizing unit
  immunoelectrophoresis
ie: *id est* (L) that is
IEA: intravascular erythrocyte aggregation
IEC:
  injection electrode catheter
  International Electrotechnical Commission
  intra-epithelial carcinoma
IEE: inner enamel epithelium
IEM: inborn error of metabolism
IEP: isolelectric point
IER test: Institute of Educational Research (intelligence) test
IF:
  immunofluorescence (test)
  inhibiting factor
  intermediate frequency
  interstitial fluid
  intrinsic factor
IFMSA: International Federation of Medical Student Associations
IFMSS: International Federation of Multiple Sclerosis Societies
If nec: if necessary
IFRP: International Fertility Research Program

IFT: International Frequency
Tables
Ig: immunoglobulin, γ-globulin
IGH: immunoreactive growth
hormone
IGY: International Geophysical
Year
IH:
infectious hepatitis
inhibiting hormone
In-patient Hospital
iron haematoxylin
IHA: indirect haemagglutination
(test)
IHD: ischaemic heart disease
IHSA: iodinated human serum
albumin
IHSS: idiopathic hypertrophic
sub-aortic stenosis
II-para: secundipara
III-para: tertipara
IJP: inhibitory junction potential
IK:
Immune Körper (Ger) immune
bodies
immunoconglutinin
I₂KI: Lugol's solution
IK unit: infusoria killing unit
IL: incisolingual
Il:
illinium (chemical symbol for)
(SEE *Pm*)
illustration
ILA:
insulin-like activity
International Leprosy Associ-
ation
ILa: incisolabial
Ileu: isoleucine
ill: illusion
illus: illustration(ed)
ILo: iodine lotion
IM:
Index Medicus
infectious mononucleosis
Internal Medicine
intramuscular(ly)
IMA:
Industrial Medical Association
Irish Medical Association
IMBI: Institute of Medical and
Biological Illustrators
immat: immature

immobil: immobilize
Immun:
immunity
immunization
Immunol: immunology
IMP: inosine monophosphate
imp:
important
impression
IMPA: incisal mandibular plane
angle
IMPS: Inpatient Multidimensional
Psychiatric Scale
Impx: impaction
IMS: Indian Medical Service
IMV: intermittent mandatory ven-
tiliation
IMViC: indol, methyl red, Voges-
Proskauer, citrate reactions
(bacteriology)
IN:
icterus neonatorum
intranasal
In:
indium (chemical symbol for)
inulin
in: inch
INA:
International Neurological
Association
Jena Nomina Anatomica (with
reference to anatomical terminology)
INAH: isonicotinic acid hydrazide
inc:
incomplete
inconclusive
incontinent
incorporated
increase(ed)(ing)
IncB: inclusion body
incompat: incompatible
incompl: incomplete
inc (R): increase (relative)
incr:
increase(ed, ing)
increment
incur: incurable
IND: Investigational New Drug
in d: *in dies* (L) daily
ind: independent
indic: indication(ed)
IndMed: Index Medicus

indust: industrial
Inf: infirmary
inf:
  infant(ile)
  infected(ion)
  inferior
  infunde (L) pour in
  infusum (L) an infusion
infect: infection(ious)
infl: influence
inflamm: inflammation(ory)
info: information
ing: inguinal
InGP: indolgylcerophosphate
INH:
  inhalation
  isoniazid
  isonicotinic acid hydrazide
  isonicotinoylhydrazine
inhib:
  inhibition
  inhibitory
INI: intranuclear inclusion (agent)
inj:
  injectable
  inject(ion)
  injury(ious)
inject: injection
inj enem: *injiciatur enema* (L) let
  an enema be injected
in litt: *in litteris* (L) in correspondence
INN: International Nonproprietary
  Names
innerv: innervation(ed)
ino: inosine
inoc: inocculation(ed)
inorg: inorganic
INPH: iproniazid phosphate
INPRONS: information processing
  in the central nervous system
in pulm: *in pulmento* (L) in gruel
INREM: internal radiation dose
ins: insurance
in situ: in natural or normal
  position
insol: insoluble
Insp: inspiration
Inspir: inspiration(atory)
Inst: institute
Instn: institution
Instr: instructor(ion)
insuff: insufficient

Int:
  intermittent
  intern, internist, internship
  internal
int cib: *inter cibos* (L) between
  meals
intell: intelligence
intern: internal
internat: international
INTEST: intestinal
INTH: intrathecal
IntMed: internal medicine
int noct: *inter noctem* (L) during
  the night
INTOX: intoxicated(-tion)
in utero: within the uterus
inv:
  inversion
  involuntary
invest: investigation
in vitro: within glass; within a test
  tube
in vivo: within a living body
invol: involuntary
I&O: intake and output
IO:
  inferior oblique (muscle)
  intestinal obstruction
  intraocular
Io: ionium (chemical symbol for)
IOC: in our culture
IOFB: intraocular foreign body
IOM: Institute of Medicine (of NAS)
IOP: intraocular pressure
IOTA: information overload testing
  aid
IP:
  icterus praecox
  incisoproximal
  incubation period
  infection prevention (with refer-
    ence to testing antiseptics)
  inpatient
  International Pharmacopia
  interphalangeal
  intraperitoneal(ly)
  iso-electric point
IPAA: International Psycho-
  analytical Association
I-para: primipara
IPC: isopropyl N-phenyl-
  carbamate
IPCS: intrauterine progesterone

contraceptive system (an IUD)

IPH: interphalangeal

IPNA: isopropylnoradrenaline

IPPA: inspection, palpation, percussion, auscultation

IPPB: intermittent positive pressure breathing

IPPB/I: intermittent positive pressure breathing/inspiratory

IPPC: isopropyl N-phenyl-carbamate (a herbicide)

IPPD: isopropyl-phenyl-paraphrenylene diamine

IPPF: International Planned Parenthood Federation

IPPR: intermittent positive pressure respiration

IPPV: intermittent positive pressure ventilation

IPQ: intimacy potential quotient

ips: inches per second

IPSP: inhibitory post-synaptic potential

IPTG: isopropyl thiogalactoside

IPU: Inpatient Unit

IPV:
inactivated poliomyelitis vaccine
infectious pustular vaginitis
infectious pustular vulvo-vaginitis (of cattle)

IQ: intelligence quotient

IR:
inferior rectus (muscle)
infra-red
internal resistance

I-R: Ito-Reenstierna (reaction)

Ir: iridium (chemical symbol for)

IRC: International Red Cross

IRGI: immunoreactive glucagon

IRI: immunoreactive insulin

IRIS: International Research Information Service

IRM:
innate releasing mechanism
Institute of Rehabilitation Medicine

IRMP: Intermountain Regional Medical Program

IRO: International Refugee Organization

IROS: ipsilateral routing of signal

IRP: International Reference Preparation

IRRG: irrigation(-ed)

IRU: Industrial Rehabilitation Unit

IRV: inspiratory reserve volume

IS:
immune serum
intercostal space
intraspinal

is: island

I-10-S: invert sugar (10%) in saline

ISA:
Instrument Society of America
iodinated serum albumin

ISADH: inappropriate secretion of antidiuretic hormone

ISC:
International Statistical Classification
interstitial cells

ISCP: International Society of Comparative Pathology

ISD: isosorbide dinitrite

ISF: interstitial fluid

ISG: immune serum globulin

ISGE: International Society of Gastroenterology

ISH: International Society of Hematology

ISI: Institute for Scientific Information

ISM: International Society of Microbiologists

ISMH: International Society of Medical Hydrology

ISO: International Standards Organization

Is of Lang: islands of Langerhans

isoln: isolation

isom: isometric

ISP:
distance between iliac spines
intraspinal

isq: *in status quo* (L) unchanged

IST: insulin shock therapy

ISU: International Society of Urology

I-substance: inhibitor substance

ISY: intrasynovial

IT:
inhalation therapy

intrathoracic
intubercular
I/T: intensity/duration
ITA:
International Tuberculosis
Association
itaconic acid
ital: italic(ize)
ITc: International Table calorie
ITh: intrathecal (intraspinal) (with
reference to injections)
ITLC: instant thin-layer
chromatography
ITP:
idiopathic thrombocytopenic
purpura
inosine triphosphate
ITR: intratracheal
ITT: insulin tolerance test
IU:
immunizing unit
international unit
intrauterine
in utero
IUB: International Union of Bio-
chemistry
IUBS: International Union of
Biological Sciences
IUFB: intrauterine foreign body
IUCD: intrauterine contraceptive
device
IUD:
intrauterine death
intrauterine device
IUGS: International Union of
Geological Sciences
IUPAC: International Union of
Pure and Applied Chemistry
IUPHAR: International Union of
Pharmacology
IUT: intrauterine transfusion
IUTM: International Union Against
Tuberculosis (*Myco-
bacterium*)
IUVDT: International Union
against Venereal Diseases
and the Treponematoses
IV:
interventricular
intervertebral
intravenous(ly)
intraventricular
iv: iodine value

IVC:
inferior vena cava
intravenous cholangiogram
IVCD: intraventricular conduction
defect
IVD: intervertebral disc
IVF: intravascular fluid
IVGTT: intravenous glucose toler-
ance test
IVJC: intervertebral joint complex
IVP:
intravenous push
intravenous pyelogram
IVPB: intravenous piggyback
IVSD: interventricular septal
defect
IVT: intravenous transfusion
I-5-W: invert sugar(5%) in water
IYS: inverted Y-suspensor
IZS: insulin zinc suspension

J

J:
Jewish
joint
journal
juice
j:
In prescription writing, used as a
Roman numeral as the equi-
valent of 'i' for *one*, *or* at the
end of a number (EX j, ij, iij, vij,
etc)
JAI: juvenile amaurotic idiocy
JAMA: Journal of the American
Medical Association
jaund: jaundice
JBE: Japanese B encephalitis
JCAE: Joint Committee on Atomic
Energy (US)
JCAH: Joint Commission on
Accreditation of Hospitals
jct: junction
JEE: Japanese equine
encephalitis
jej: jejunum
jentac: *jentaculum* (L) breakfast
JFS: Jewish Family Service
JG: juxtaglomerular
JGA: juxtaglomerular apparatus

JH: juvenile hormone (of insects)
JHMO: Junior Hospital Medical Officer
JJ: jaw jerk
JNA: Jena Nomina Anatomica (SEE *INA*)
JND: just noticeable difference
jnt: joint
Jour: journal
JPSA: Joint Program for the Study of Abortions
JS unit: Junkman-Schoeller unit (of thyrotrophin)
jt: joint
jucund: *jucunde* (L) pleasantly
juv: juvenile
JV: jugular vein
JVP: jugular vein pulse

K

K:
  absolute zero
  electrostatic capacity
  capsular antigen (from Kapsel)
  ionization constant
  Kelvin (temperature scale)
  potassium (L) *kalium* (chemical symbol for)
k:
  constant
  kilo (prefix)
  a thousand
κ: kappa (tenth letter of the Greek alphabet)
K-10: gastric tube
17-K: 17-ketosteroids
KA:
  alkaline phosphatase
  ketoacidosis
  King-Armstrong (units)
ka: kathode (cathode)
KAAD mixture: kerosene, alcohol, acetic acid, dioxane mixture (for killing insect larvae)
Kal: *kalium* (L) potassium
KAP: knowledge, aptitude, and practices (with reference to fertility)
K/A ratio: ratio of ketogenic to

antiketogenic substances (in diets)
kat: katal (enzyme unit)
KAU: King-Armstrong unit
KB: ketone bodies
KC: kathodal (cathodal) closing
kc: kilocycle
Kcal: kilocalorie (1000 calories)
KCC: kathodal (cathodal) closing contraction
kcps: kilocycles per second
kc/s: kilocycles per second
KCT: kathodal (cathodal) closing tetanus
KD: kathodal (cathodal) duration
KDT: kathodal (cathodal) duration tetanus
KE:
  Kendall's compound E (cortisone)
  kinetic energy
K_e: exchangeable body potassium
keto: 17-ketosteroid test
kev: kiloelectron volts
kf: symbol indicating flocculation speed in antigen-antibody reactions
KFD: Kyasanur Forest disease (of South India)
kg: kilogram
kg-cal: kilocalorie (large calorie)
kg-m: kilogram-metre
kgps: kilogram per second
KGS: ketogenic steroid
17-KGS: 17-ketogenic steroids
KHb: potassium haemoglobinate (chemical formula for)
kHz: kilohertz
KI:
  Krönig's isthmus
  potassium iodide (chemical formula for)
KIA: Kligler iron agar (medium)
kilo: a thousand
KIU: Kallikrein inhibiting unit
KJ: knee jerk
KK: knee kick (knee jerk)
kl:
  kilolitre
  Klang (Ger) a compound musical overtone
KL bac: Klebs-Loeffler bacillus (diphtheria bacillus)

Klebs: *Klebsiella*
KLH: keyhole limpet haemocyanin
KLS: kidney, liver, spleen
Km: Michaelis constant
km: kilometre
kMc: kilomegacycle
KMEF: keratin, myosin, epidermin, fibrin (class of proteins)
kmps: kilometres per sec
KNL: Darrow's solution (for anti-diarrhoea potassium therapy)
KO: knocked out
KOC: kathodal (cathodal) opening contraction
KP:
  keratic precipitates
  keratitis punctata
K-P: Kaiser-Permanente (diet)
KPI: karyopyknotic index
Kr: krypton (chemical symbol for)
KRP: Kolmer test with Reiter protein
KS: ketosteroid
17-KS: 17-ketosteroids
KSC: kathodal (cathodal) closing contraction
KSCN: potassium thiocyanate (broth)
KST: kathodal (cathodal) closing tetanus
K stoff: chloromethyl chloroformate (a war gas)
KTSA: Kahn Test of Symbol Arrangement
KUB:
  kidney and upper bladder
  kidney, ureter, and bladder
kv: kilovolt
kva: kilovolt-ampere
kvcp: kilovolt constant potential
kvp: kilovolts peak
kw: kilowatt
kw-hr: kilowatt-hour

L

L:
  Avogadro's constant
  coefficient of induction
  Lactobacillus
  Lambert (a unit of light)

  Latin
  left
  lethal
  lewisite
  liber (L) book
  libra (L) pound
  licensed to practice
  light
  light (chain of protein molecules)
  light sense
  lilac (an indicator colour)
  lime
  lingual
  low (when followed by another abbr., e.g. LBP)
  lower(est)
  Heat labile component of protein antigen of vaccinia and variola viruses
l:
  laevorotatory
  left
  left eye
  length
  lethal
  litre
  long
  longitudinal (with reference to sections)
  lumen
λ: lambda (eleventh letter of the Greek alphabet)
L-: laevorotatory
L_1, L_2: first lumbar vertebra, second lumbar vertebra, etc
L/3: lower third (with reference to long bones)
L_+: limes death; *limes tod*
L_o: limes zero; *limes nul*
l-: laevo- (or counterclockwise) (in chemical formula)
LA:
  left angle(ation) (orthopaedics)
  left atrium
  left auricle
  leucine aminopeptidase
  linguo-axial
  local anaesthesia
  long-acting (with reference to drugs)
L&A: light and accommodation (with reference to reaction of pupils)

La:
  labial
  lanthanum (chemical symbol
    for)
la: *lege artis* (L) according to the
  art
LAAO: L-amino acid oxidase
lab:
  laboratory
  rennet (Ger)
lab proc: laboratory procedure
LABS: Laboratory Admission
  Baseline Studies
LAC: linguo-axiocervical
LaC: labiocervical
lac: laceration(s)
LAD:
  lactic acid dehydrogenase
  left axis deviation
LADA: left-acromio-
    dorso-anterior (position of
    fetus)
LADP: left-acromio-dorso-
    posterior (position of fetus)
LAE: left atrial enlargement
laev: *laevus* (L) left
LAF: laminar air flow
LAG: linguo-axiogingival
LaG: labiogingival
lag: *lagena* (L) flask, bottle
LAH: Licentiate of Apothecaries
  Hall, Dublin
Lal: labioincisal
LAIT: latex agglutination inhibition
  test (for pregnancy)
LaL: labiolingual
lam: laminectomy
LAO: Licentiate of the Art of
  Obstetrics
LAP:
  leucine aminopeptidase
  leukocyte alkaline phosphatase
  lyophilized anterior pituitary
lap: laparotomy
lapid: *lapideum* (L) stony
LAR: laryngology
lar: left arm reclining or recumbent
LARC: leucocyte automatic
  recognition computer
Laryngol: laryngology(ist)
LAS:
  linear alkyl sulfonate
  local adaptation syndrome

LASER: light amplification by
  stimulated emission of
  radiation
lat: lateral
lat admov: *lateri admoveatum* (L)
  let it be applied to the side
lat dol: *lateri dolenti* (L) to the painful side
LATS: long-acting thyroid
  stimulator
LB: low back (disorder)
L&B: left and below
lb: *libra* (L) pound
LBBsB: left bundle branch system
  block
LBCD: left border cardiac dull-
  ness
LBCF: Laboratory Branch
  Complement Fixation (test)
LBD: left border of dullness (of
  heart to percussion)
LBF: *Lactobacillus bulgaricus*
  factor (pantetheine)
LBH: length, breadth, height
LBM: lean body mass
LBP:
  low back pain
  low blood pressure
LC: linguocervical
LCA: left coronary artery
LCAT: lecithin-cholesterol acetyl-
  transferase
LCCS: low cervical Caesarean
  section
LCFA: long chain fatty acid
LCh: Licentiate in Surgery
LCL: Levinthal-Coles-Lillie
  (bodies)
LCM:
  left costal margin
  lowest common multiple
  lymphocytic choriomeningitis
LCME: Liaison Committee on
  Medical Education
LCP: long chain polysaturated
  (fatty acids)
LCPS: Licentiate of the College of
  Physicians and Surgeons
LD:
  lactic dehydrogenase
  lethal dose
  light-dark
  light difference, perception of

linguodistal
living donor
low density
LD$_{50}$: median lethal dose
LDA: left dorso-anterior (position of fetus)
LDE: lauric diethamide
LDH: lactate dehydrogenase
LDL: low-density lipoprotein
LDP: left dorsoposterior (position of fetus)
LDS: Licentiate in Dental Surgery
LDSc: Licentiate in Dental Science
LDUB: long double upright brace
LE:
  left eye
  lower extremity
  lupus erythematosus
Le: Leonard (unit for cathode rays)
Lect: lecturer
leg: legal(ly)
leg com: legally committed
LEM: Leibovitz-Emory (medium)
lenit: *leniter* (L) gently
LEP: low egg passage (strain of virus)
Lept: *Leptospira*
LES:
  local excitatory state
  Locke egg serum (medium)
  lower esophageal sphincter
LET: lineal energy transfer
Leu: leucine
lev: *levis* (L) light
l/ext: lower extremity
L$_f$: flocculation units (of toxin per ml)
Lf: limit of flocculation
lf: low frequency
LFA: left fronto-anterior (left mentoanterior) (position of fetus)
LFD:
  least fatal dose (of a toxin)
  low-fat diet
LFH: left femoral hernia
LFP: left frontoposterior (left mentoposterior) (position of fetus)
LFPS: Licentiate of the Faculty of Physicians and Surgeons
LFT:
  latex fixation test

left frontotransverse (left mentotransverse) (position of fetus)
liver function tests
low frequency transduction
LG: linguogingival
lg: large
lge: large
LGH: lactogenic hormone
LGV: lymphogranuloma venereum
LH:
  left hand
  left hyperphoria
  lower half
  lues hereditaria
  luteinizing hormone (ICSH)
LHC: left hypochondrium
l-hr: lumen hour
LHRF: luteinizing hormone releasing factor
LHS:
  left hand side
  left heart strain
LHT: left hypertropia
LI: linguoincisal
LI, LII, LIII: (SEE *lues*)
Li: lithium (chemical symbol for)
lib: *libra* (L) pound
LIBC: latent iron-binding capacity
LIC: limiting isorrhoeic concentration
Lic: Licentiate
LICM: left intercostal margin
LicMed: Licentiate in Medicine
LIF:
  left iliac fossa
  leucocytosis-inducing factor
lig: ligament
LIH: left inguinal hernia
lim: limit
lin: linear
linim: liniment
Linn: Linnaeus(an)
Lip:
  lipoate (lipoic acid)
  liquor (L) a liquor or liquid
liq: liquid
LIRBM: liver, iron, red bone marrow
LIS: lobular in situ (carcinoma)
lit: literal(ly)

LIV:
  law of initial value (Joseph Wilder)
  liver battery test (dentistry)
LKQCPI: Licentiate of the King and Queen's College of Physicians in Ireland
LKS: liver, kidney, spleen
LL:
  left lower
  lower lid
LLBCD: left lower border of cardiac dullness
LLD factor: Lactobacillus lactis Dorner factor (vitamin B_{12})
LLE: left lower extremity
LLF:
  Laki-Lorand factor (fibrinase)
  left lateral femoral (site of injection)
LLL:
  left lower eyelid
  left lower lobe (of lung)
LLM: localized leukocyte mobilization
LLQ: left lower quadrant (of abdomen)
LM:
  legal medicine
  Licentiate in Medicine
  Licentiate in Midwifery
  light minimum
  linguomesial
  lipid mobilizing (hormone)
  longitudinal muscle
  lower motor (neuron)
lm: lumen
LMA: left mentoanterior (position of fetus)
LMCC: Licentiate of the Medical Council of Canada
LMD: local medical doctor
LMedLCh: Licentiate in Medicine and Surgery
LML: left mediolateral (with reference to episiotomy)
LMM: light meromyosin
LMN: lower motor neuron
LMNL: lower motor neuron lesion
LMP:
  last menstrual period

  left mentoposterior (position of fetus)
  lumbar puncture
LMRCP: Licentiate in Midwifery of the Royal College of Physicians
LMS: Licentiate in Medicine and Surgery
LMSSA: Licentiate in Medicine and Surgery of the Society of Apothecaries, London
LMT: left mentotransverse (position of fetus)
ln: logarithm, natural
LNMP: last normal menstrual period
LNPF: lymph node permeability factor
LO: linguo-occlusal
LOA:
  leave of absence
  left occipito-anterior (position of fetus)
lo cal: low calorie (diet)
lo calc: low calcium (diet)
loc cit: *loco citato* (L) in the place quoted
loc dol: *loco dolenti* (L) to the painful spot
log: logarithm
log$_e$: logarithm to the base e
log$_{10}$: logarithm to the base 10
LOL: left occipitolateral (position of fetus)
LOM: limitation of movement or motion
LOMSA: left otitis media suppurative acute
LOMSCh: left otitis media suppurative chronic
long: longitudinal
LOP:
  leave on pass
  left occipitoposterior (position of fetus)
LOPS: length of patient stay
lord: lordosis (tic)
LOS:
  length of stay
  Licentiate in Obstetrical Science
LOT: left occipitotransverse (position of fetus)

lot: *lotio* (L) lotion
LP:
  laboratory procedure
  latent period
  light perception
  linguopulpal
  lipoprotein
  low power (with reference to microscopy)
  low pressure
  lumbar puncture
L/P:
  lactate/pyruvate (ratio)
  lymphocyte/polymorph (ratio)
LPF:
  leucocytosis-promoting factor
  low-power field
LPH: lipotrophic pituitary hormone (lipotrophin)
LPL: lipoprotein lipase
LPN: Licensed Practical Nurse
lps: litres per second
lpw: lumens per watt
LQ: lowest quadrant
LR:
  laboratory report
  latency relaxation
  lateral rectus (muscle)
Lr: lawrencium (chemical symbol for)
LRCP: Licentiate of the Royal College of Physicians
LRCP&SI: Licentiate of the Royal College of Physicians and Surgeons, Ireland
LRCS: Licentiate of the Royal College of Surgeons
LRCSE: Licentiate of the Royal College of Surgeons, Edinburgh
LRCSI: Licentiate of the Royal College of Surgeons, Ireland
LRF:
  latex and resorcinol formaldehyde
  liver residue factor
  luteinizing hormone-releasing factor
LRFPS: Licentiate of the Royal Faculty of Physicians and Surgeons
LRH: luteinizing hormone-releasing hormone

LRL: Lunar Receiving Laboratory
LRR: labyrinthine righting reflex
LS:
  lateral suspensor
  Licentiate in Surgery
  liminal sensitivity
  lumbosacral
LSA:
  left sacro-anterior (position of fetus)
  Licentiate of the Society of Apothecaries, London
LSB: left sternal border
LSC: liquid scintillation counting
LScA: left scapulo-anterior (position of fetus)
LScP: left scapuloposterior (position of fetus)
LSCS: lower segment Caesarean section
LSD:
  League for Spiritual Discovery
  least significant difference
LSD 25: *d*-lysergic acid diethylamine tartrate 25 (a hallucinogen)
LSH: lymphocyte-stimulating hormone (factor)
LSI: large scale integrated (circuit)
LSK: liver, spleen, kidneys
LSL: left sacrolateral (position of fetus)
LSM: lysergic acid morpholide
LSP: left sacroposterior (position of fetus)
LSp: life span
LST: left sacrotransverse (position of fetus)
LSU: lactose-saccharose-urea (agar)
LT:
  low temperature
  lymphotoxin
lt:
  left
  low tension
LTAS: lead tetra-acetate Schiff
LTB: laryngotracheal bronchitis
LTC: long term care
ltd: limited
LTF:
  lipotropic factor
  lymphocyte transforming factor

LTH:
low-temperature holding
(pasteurization)
luteotrophic hormone
LTPP: lipothiamide-pyro-
phosphate
LTT: lymphocyte transformation
test
LU: left upper
Lu: lutetium (chemical symbol
for)
LUE: left upper extremity
Lues I: primary syphilis
Lues II: secondary syphilis
Lues III: tertiary syphilis
LUL:
left upper eyelid
left upper lobe (of lung)
LUO: left ureteral orifice
LUOQ: left upper outer quandrant
LUQ: left upper quadrant (of
abdomen)
lut: *luteum* (L) yellow
LV:
left ventricle
live vaccine
Lv: leave
LVED: left ventricular end dia-
stolic
LVH: left ventricular hypertrophy
LVLG: left ventrolateral gluteal
(site of injection)
LVN:
Licensed Visiting Nurse
Licensed Vocational Nurse
LVS: left ventricular strain
LVT: lysine vasotonin
Lw: lawrencium
L&W: living and well
L-10-W: laevulose (10%) in water
LY: lactoalbumin-yeastolate (with
reference to bacteriological
media)
ly: Langley (unit of sun's heat)
lym: lymphocyte
lymph: lymphocyte
lymphos: lymphocytes
Lys: lysine
lytes: electrolytes
LZM: lysozyme

M

M:
macerare (L) macerate
male
malignant (with reference to
tumours)
married
mass
massage
mature
maximal (mum)
mean (arithmetic)
median
mediator (chemical, released in
the tissues)
medical
mega (prefix)
memory (associative)
mentum (L) chin
meridies (L) noon
mesial
metabolite
Micrococcus
mille (L) thousand
misce (L) mix
mistura (L) mixture
mitte (L) send
molar (solution)
molar (tooth, permanent)
molecular weight
Monday
monkey
morphine
mother
motile (with reference to
bacteria)
mucoid (with reference to
bacterial colonies)
murmur (heart)
muscle
mutitas (L) dullness
myopia
m:
manipulus (L) handful
melts at (when followed by
a figure denoting temperature)
metre
milli (prefix)
minim

minute
molar (tooth, deciduous)
murmur

μ:
micro (prefix)
mu (twelfth letter of Greek
alphabet)
symbol for micron

m-:
meta- (in chemical formulas)
prefix denoting meso-position

M₁, M₂, M₃: Slight, marked, and
absolute dullness (aus-
cultation)

M₁: mitral (first) sound
M₂: dose per square metre of body
surface
M/3: middle third (long bones)

MA:
Master of Arts
menstrual age
mental age
mentum anterior
meter angle

ma: milliampere

MAA:
macroaggregated albumin
Medical Assistance to the Aged

MAAGB: Medical Artists
Association of Great Britain

MABP: mean arterial blood
pressure

MAC:
malignancy associated changes
maximal allowable concentration
maximal allowable cost

mac: *macerare* (L) macerate
m accur: *misce accuratissme (L)*
mix very intimately
macer: *macera* (L) macerate

MAD:
methylandrostenediol
mind-altering drug

MAF: minimum audible field
Mag: magnesium

mag:
magnification
magnus (L) large

Magic: microprobe analysis
generalized intensity correc-
tions

magn: *magnus* (L) large

Mal: malate
M+Am: compound myopic
astigmatism
ma-min: milliampere-minute

man:
mane (L) morning
manipulus (L) a handful

mand: mandible
manifest: manifestation
manip: *manipulus* (L) a handful
man pr: *mane primo* (L) early in
the morning
manuf: manufacture

MAO:
Master of the Art of Obstetrics
monoamine oxidase

MAOI: monoamine oxidase
inhibitor
MAOT: Member of the Association
of Occupational Therapists

MAP:
mean arterial pressure
Medical Audit Program
minimum audible pressure
muscle action potential

MAR: minimal angle resolution
MAS: milliampere-second
mas: masculine
masc: masculine
MASER: microwave amplification
by stimulated emission of
radiation
mas pil: *massa pilularum* (L) a pill
mass
mass: massage
mast: mastoid
MASU: Mobile Army Surgical Unit
MAT: manual arts therapist
math: mathematics(ical)
matut: *matutinus* (L) in the
morning

max:
maxilla
maximum

MB:
buccal margin
Marsh-Bender factor (an ATP
inhibitor in muscle tissue)
Medicinae Baccalaureus (L)
Bachelor of Medicine
mesiobuccal
methyl bromide
methylene blue

mb: *misce bene* (L) mix well

MBAC: Member of the British Association of Chemists

MBC: maximum breathing capacity

MBD: minimal brain dysfunction

MB factor: Marsh-Bender factor

MBH₂: methylene blue reduced

MBL:
Marine Biological Laboratory (Woods Hole, Mass)
menstrual blood loss

MBO: mesiobucco-occlusal

MBP:
mean blood pressure
melitensis, bovine, porcine
mesiobuccupulpal

MBRT: methylene blue reduction time

MC:
Magister Chirurgiae (L) Master of Surgery
Medical Corps
mesiocervical
metacarpal
monkey cells
myocarditis

M-C:
Medico-Chirurgical
mineralocorticoid (with reference to adrenal cortical hormones)

M&C: morphine and cocaine

Mc:
megacurie
megacycle

mc: millicurie

MCA: Manufacturing Chemists Association

MCAT: Medical College Admission Test

m caute: *misce caute*: (L) mix cautiously

MCB: membranous cytoplasmic bodies

McB: McBurney's (point)

MCC: marked cocontraction

McC: McCarthy (panendoscope)

MCCU: Mobile Coronary Care Unit

MCD: mean corpuscular diameter

mcd: millicuries destroyed

MCF: medium corpuscular fragility

mcg: microgram

MCH:
Maternal and Child Health
mean corpuscular haemoglobin

MCh: *Margister Chirurgiae* (L) Master of Surgery

mc h: millicurie hour

MCHC: mean corpuscular haemoglobin concentration

MChD: Master of Dental Surgery

MChir: Master in Surgery

MChOrth: Master of Orthopaedic Surgery

MCHR: Medical Committee for Human Rights

MChS: Member of the Society of Chiropodists

MCi: megacurie

mCi: millicurie

MCL:
midclavicular line
modified chest lead

mcoul: millicoulomb

μ **coul:** microcoulomb

MCP: metacarpophalangeal

MCPA: Member of the College of Pathologists, Australasia

MCPH: metacarpophalangeal

MCPS: Member of the College of Physicians & Surgeons

Mcps: megacycles per second

MCR:
Medical Corps Reserve
metabolic clearance rate

MCRA: Member of the College of Radiologists, Australasia

MCSP: Member of the Chartered Society of Physiotherapists

MCT:
mean circulation time
medium chain triglyceride
multiple compressed tablet

MCTD:
mixed connective tissue disease

MCV: mean corpuscular volume

MCZ: Museum of Comparative Zoology (Harvard Univ)

MD:
malic dehydrogenase
manic-depressive
mean deviation
Medical Department
Medicinae Doctor (L) Doctor of Medicine

mentally deficient
mesiodistal
mitral disease
muscular dystrophy
myocardial disease

Md: mendelevium (chemical symbol)

md: median

MDA:
mento-dextra anterior (L) right mento-anterior (position of fetus)
monodehydroascorbate
motor discriminative acuity
Muscular Dystrophy Association

MDCK: Madin-Darby-canine kidney (cell line)

MDD: Doctor of Dental Medicine

MDentSc: Master of Dental Science

MDF: myocardial depressant factor

MDH: malic dehydrogenase

m dict: *more dictu* (L) in the manner directed

mdn: median

MDNB: metadinitrobenzene

MDP: *mento-dextra posterior* (L) right mentoposterior (position of fetus)

MDQ: minimum detectable quantity

MDR: minimum daily requirement

MDS: Master of Dental Surgery

MDT: *mento-dextra transversa* (L) right mentotransverse (position of fetus)

ME:
maximum effort
median eminence (of hypothalamus)
Medical Examiner
metabolizable energy
middle ear

M/E: myeloid/erythrocyte (ratio)

Me: methyl (CH_3)

MEA:
mercaptoethyl amine
multiple endocrine adenomas

meas: measure(ment)

MeB: methylene blue

MEC: minimum effective concentration

mec: meconium

Mecano: mechanotherapy

mech: mechanical

MED:
median erythrocyte diameter
medical
medicine
minimal effective dose
minimal erythema dose

med:
median(al)
medical
medication
medicine(al)
medium (bacteriology)

MEDEX: *medecin extension* (F) extension of the physician (with reference to recruitment program)

MEDICO: Medical International Cooperation

MEDLARS: Medical Literature Analysis and Retrieval System

MEDLINE: an on-line segment of MEDLARS

MEDScD: Doctor of Medical Science

Med Tech:
Medical Technician
Medical Technology(ist)

MEE: methylethyl ether

MEF: maximal expiratory flow

meg: megacycle

MEM: minimum essential medium

mem: member

memb: membrane

MEND: Medical Education for National Defense

Menn: Menninger

ment: mental

MeOH: methyl alcohol

MEP:
mean effective pressure
motor end-plate

MEPP: miniature end-plate potential

mEq: milliequivalent

MER: ethamoxytriphetol (an anti-oestrogen)

Mer-29: triparanol (an anti-cholesterol drug)

MES: maintenance electrolyte solution

Mesc: mescaline
Met: methionine
met: metallic (with reference to chest sounds)
metab: metabolism(ic)
metaph: metaphysics
metas: metastasize (sis)
Meth: methedrine
meth: methyl
MeThCh: methylthiocholine
M et n: *mane et nocte* (L) morning and night
m et sig: *misce et signa* (L) mix and write a label
mev: million electron volts
MF:
  microscopic factor
  mitotic figure
  multiplying factor
  mycosis fungoides
M/F: male to female (ratio)
Mf: *Microfilaria*
μ**f:** microfarad
mf: millifarad
MFA: methyl fluoracetate
MFD: minimum fatal dose
mfd: microfarad
MFG: modified heat degraded gelatin (a plasma extender)
mfg: manufacturing(ed)
MFHom: Member of the Faculty of Homeopathy
M flac: *membrana flaccida* (L) Shrapnell's membrane
MF method: membrane or millipore filter method (bacteriology)
mfr: manufacturer
MF sol: merthiolate-formaldehyde (stock) solution (SEE *MIF*)
MFT: muscle function test
m ft: *mistura fiat* (L) let a mixture be made
MG:
  margin
  menopausal gonadotrophin
  mesiogingival
  myasthenia gravis
Mg: magnesium (chemical symbol for)
mg: milligram
mg%: milligrams per 100 ml
μ**g:** microgram

MGA: melengestrol acetate (a progestin)
MGD: mixed gonadal dysgenesis
mgd: million gallons per day
mg-el: milligram element
MGH: Massachusetts General Hospital
mgh: milligram-hour
mgm: milligram
MGP: marginal granulocyte pool
MGW: magnesium sulphate, glycerine, water (enema)
MH:
  mammotrophic hormone (prolactin)
  marital history
  medical history
  melanophore hormone
  menstrual history
  mental health
mh: millihenry
MHA: Mental Health Administration
MHb: myohaemoglobin
mhcb: mean horizontal candle power
MHD:
  magnetohydrodynamics
  minimum haemolytic dose
MHPG: methoxyhydroxy-phenylglycol
MHRI: Mental Health Research Institute (Univ of Michigan)
MH virus: murine hepatitis virus
MHyg: Master of Hygiene
MHz: megahertz
MI:
  mesioincisal
  metabolic index
  mitral incompetence
  mitral insufficiency
  myocardial infarction
MIBT: methyl isatin-beta-thiosemicarbasone
MIC:
  minimal inhibitory concentration
  minimal isorrhoeic concentration
mic:
  microscopic findings in centrifuged urinary sediment
  microscopy(ic)
Microbiol: microbiology

MICU: Mobile Intensive Care Unit
MID:
   mesioincisodistal
   minimal inhibiting dose
   minimum infective dose
mid: middle
mid sag: midsagittal
MIF:
   melanocyte-stimulating hor-
      mone release-inhibiting factor
   merthiolate-iodine-formaldehyde
      (technique for faecal examin-
      ation)
   migration-inhibitory factor (for
      macrophages)
MIFR: maximal inspiratory flow
      rate
mil: military
MIMS: Monthly Index of Medical
      Specialities
min:
   mineral
   minimum (L) a minim
   minimum(al)
   minor
   minute
MINA: monoisonitrosoacetone
MINIA: monkey intranuclear inclu-
      sion agent
MInstSP: Member Institution of
      Sewage Purification
MIO: minimal identifiable odour
misc:
   miscarriage
   miscellaneous
MIST: Medical Information Service
      by Telephone
mist: *mistura* (L) a mixture
MIT:
   Massachusetts Institute of
      Technology
   miracidial immobilization test
   mono-iodotyrosine
mit: *mitte* (L) send
mit insuf: mitral insufficiency
mitt: *mitte* (L) send
mitte sang: *mitte sanguinem* (L)
      bleed
mitt tal: *mitte tales* (L) send such
mixt: *mixture* (L) mixture
MJ: marijuana
MK: monkey kidney
mkg: metre kilogram

mks: metre-kilogram-second
ML:
   Licentiate in Medicine
   lingual margin
   mesiolingual
   midline
mL: millilambert
ml: millilitre (1/1000 of a litre)
MLA:
   Medical Library Association
   mento-laeva anterior (L) left
      mento-anterior (position of
      fetus)
MLa: mesiolabial
MLaI: mesiolabioincisal
MLaP: mesiolabiopulpal
MLC: mixed leucocyte culture
MLD:
   metachromatic leucodystrophy
   minimal lethal dose
MLD 50: median lethal dose
      (radiation)
MLI: mesiolinguoincisal
MLO: mesiolinguo-occlusal
MLP:
   mento-laeva posterior (L) left
      mento-posterior (position of
      fetus)
   mesiolinguopulpal
MLS:
   median life span
   median longitudinal section
MLT:
   median lethal time (radiation)
   Medical Laboratory Technician
   mento-laeva transversa (L) left
      mentotransverse (position of
      fetus)
MM:
   Major Medical (insurance)
   mucous membrane
   myeloid metaplasia
mM: millimolar
mm:
   millimetre
   muscles
MMA: methyl malonic acid
MMD: mass median diameter (of
      particles)
MMDA: trimethoxyamphetamine
MMED: Master of Medicine
MMEFR: maximum mid-
      expiratory flow rate

MMF:
  maximum midexpiratory flow (rate)
  Member of the Medical Faculty
mmHg: millimetres of mercury
MMIS: Medicade Management and Information System
mmm: millimicron (nanometer)
MMPI: Minnesota Multiphasic Personality Inventory
mmpp: millimetres partial pressure
MMR:
  Mass Miniature Radiography
  maternal mortality rate
  monomethylolrutin
MMS: Master of Medical Science
mm st: muscle strength
MMT: manual muscle test
MMTV: mouse mammary tumour virus
MMU: mercaptomethyl uracil
mmu: millimass units
mμ: millimicron (nanometer)
mμc: millimicrocurie (nanocurie)
mμg: millimicrogram (nanogram)
μl: microlitre
μmg: micromilligram
μmm: micromillimetre
$\mu\mu$: micromicron (picometer)
$\mu\mu$c: micromicrocurie (picocurie)
$\mu\mu$g: micromicrogram (pico-gram)
MN:
  mononuclear (leucocyte)
  motor neuron
  multinodular
  myoneural
Mn: manganese (chemical symbol for)
mN: millinormal (1/1000 of normal)
MND: minimum necrosing dose
mng: morning
MNJ: myoneural junction
MO:
  manually operated
  Medical Officer
  mesio-occlusal
  mineral oil
  minute output (of heart)
  molecular orbit (contour)

Mo:
  mode
  molybdenum (chemical symbol for)
mo: month
mob: mobilization
mobil: mobility
MOD: mesio-occlusodistal
mod: moderate
mod praesc: *modo praescripto* (L) in the manner prescribed or as directed
MOF: marine oxidation/fermentation (medium)
MO&G: Master of Obstetrics and Gynaecology
MOH: Medical Officer of Health
MΩ: megohm
$\mu\Omega$: microhm
mol: molecule(ar)
mol/l: molecules per litre
moll: *mollis* (L) soft
mol wt: molecular weight
MOM: milk of magnesia
Mon: Monday
mon: monocyte
Mono: mononucleosis
mono: monocyte
MOPV: monovalent oral poliovirus vaccine
MORC: Medical Officers Reserve Corps
mor dict: *more dicto* (L) in the manner directed
morph: morphology(ical)
mor sol: *more solito* (L) in the usual manner
mortal: mortality
mos: months
mOsm: milliosmol
MOTT: mycobacteria other than tubercle (bacilli)
MP:
  menstrual period
  mentum posterior
  mesiopulpal
  metacarpophalangeal (with reference to joints of the hand
  metatarsophalangeal (with reference to joints of the foot)
  mucopolysaccharide
mp: melting point

6-MP: mercaptopurine (an anti-cancer agent)

MPB: male pattern baldness

MPC: maximum permissible concentration

MPCU: maximum permissible concentration of unidentified radio-nucleotides

MPD:
maximum permissible dose
myofacial pain dysfunction

MPH: Master of Public Health

mph: miles per hour

MPharm: Master in Pharmacy

MPI:
maximum point of impulse
multiphasic personality inventory

MPL: maximum permissible level

MPM: multipurpose meal

MPN: most probable number

MPR: marrow production rate

MPS:
Member of the Pharmaceutical Society
movement produced stimuli
mucopolysaccharide
multiphasic screening

MPU: Medical Practitioners Union

MR:
may repeat
medial rectus (muscle)
mentally retarded
metabolic rate
methyl red (as indicator)

mR: milliroentgen

μR: microroentgen

MRA: Medical Record Administrator

MRACP: Member of Royal Australian College of Physicians

MRad: Master of Radiology

mrad: millirad

MRBC: monkey red blood cells

MRC:
Medical Registration Council
Medical Research Council
Medical Reserve Corps
methylrosaniline chloride

MRCGP: Member of the Royal College of General Practitioners

MRCI:
Medical Registration Council of Ireland
Medical Research Council of Ireland

MRCOG: Member of the Royal College of Obstetricians and Gynaecologists

MRCP: Member of the Royal College of Physicians

MRCPE: Member of the Royal College of Physicians of Edinburgh

MRCP(Glasg): Member of the Royal College of Physicians and Surgeons of Glasgow *qua* Physician

MRCPI: Member of the Royal College of Physicians of Ireland

MRCS: Member of the Royal College of Surgeons

MRCSE: Member of the Royal College of Surgeons of Edinburgh

MRCSI: Member of the Royal College of Surgeons in Ireland

MRCVS: Member of the Royal College of Veterinary Surgeons

MRD: minimum reaction dose

mrd: millirutherford

mrem: milliroentgen equivalent man

mrep: milliroentgen equivalent physical

MRF: MSH releasing factor

MRH: MSH-releasing hormone

mrhm: milliroentgen per hour at one metre

MRI: Member of the Royal Institution

MRL: Medical Record Librarian

mRNA: messenger ribonucleic acid

MRR: marrow release rate

MRSH: Member of the Royal Society of Health

MRU:
Mass Radiography Unit
minimal reproductive units (bacteriology)

MRV: mixed respiratory vaccine

MRVP: methyl red, Voges-Proskauer (medium)

MS:
complex of substrate and activating metal ion
mass spectrometry
Master of Science
Master of Surgery
mentally retarded
mitral stenosis
modal sensitivity
molar solution
morphine sulphate
multiple sclerosis
muscle shortening
muscle strength
musculoskeletal

Ms: manuscript

MS-222: tricaine methane sulphonate

MSA:
manitol salt agar (plate)
Medical Services Administration
mine safety appliance

MSC: Medical Service Corps

MSc: Master of Science

mscp: mean spherical candle power

MSDC: Mass Spectrometry Data Centre (UK)

mse: mean square error

msec: millisecond

μ**sec:** microsecond

MSG: monosodium glutamate

MSH:
melanocyte-stimulating hormone
melanophore-stimulating hormone (intermedin)

MSH-IF: MSH-inhibiting factor

MSL: midsternal line

MSN: Master of Science in Nursing

MSPH: Master of Science in Public Health

MSR: Member of the Society of Radiographers

MSRG: Member of the Society for Remedial Gymnasts

MSRPP: multidimensional scale for rating psychiatric patients

MSS:
massage

Medical Superintendents' Society
mental status schedule

Mss: manuscripts

MSSE: Master of Science in Sanitary Engineering

MSSVD: Medical Society for the Study of Venereal Diseases

MST: mean survival time

MSTh: mesothorium

MSU: mid-stream urine specimen

MSUD: maple syrup urine disease

MSurg: Master of Surgery

MSV: murine sarcoma virus

MSW:
Master of Social Welfare
Master of Social Work
Medical Social Worker

MT:
empty
Medical Technologist
membrana tympani
metatarsal
music therapy

MT6: mercaptomerin (Thiomerin)

MTA: Medical Technical Assistant

MT(ASCP): Registered Medical Technologist (American Society of Clinical Pathologists)

MTD: Midwife Teacher's Diploma

mtd: *mitte tales doses* (L) send such doses

MTP: metatarsophalangeal

MTR: Meinicke turbidity reaction

MTT: mean transit time (SEE *TT*)

MTU: methylthiouracil

M tuberc: *Mycobacterium tuberculosis*

MTV: mammary tumour virus

MTX: methotrexate

MU: mouse unit (with reference to gonadotrophins)

Mu: Mache unit (with reference to radium emanations)

mu: micron (μ)

μ**U:** microunit

MUC: maximum urinary concentratrion

muc: *mucilago (L)* mucilage

mult: multiple

MuLV: murine leukaemia virus

MUO: myocardiopathy of
unknown origin
MurNAc: N-acetylmuramate
musc: muscle(ular)
MUWU: mouse uterine weight unit
MV:
Medicus Veterinarius (L)
veterinary physician
microvilli
microwave
minute volume
mitral valve
Mv: mendelevium (chemical
symbol for)
mV: millivolt
μ**V:** microvolt
MVE: Murray Valley encephalitis
MVRI: mixed vaccine, respiratory
infections
MVV: maximum voluntary
ventilation
MW: molecular weight
μ**w:** microwatt
Mx: Medix
My: myopia
my: mayer (a unit of heat capacity)
Myco: *Mycobacterium*
Mycol: mycology
Myel: myelocyte
myel: myelin(ated)
MyG: myasthenia gravis
MZ: monozygotic

N

N:
nasal
negative
negro
nerve
neurology(ist)
nicotinamide
nitrogen (chemical symbol)
non-malignant (with reference
to tumours)
Nonne (globulin test)
normal (with reference to
solutions: 2N equals twice
normal, N/2 or 0.5N equals
one-half normal, 0.1N equals
one-tenth normal)
normal (with reference to
structure and function-
ing of organs)
number
n:
born
symbol for index of refraction
haploid chromosome number
(2n equals diploid number)
nano (prefix)
naris (L) nostril
nasal
natus (L) born
neuter
neutron
neutron dosage (unit of)
number
symbol (chemical) for normal
N: radioactive nitrogen
NI, NII, etc: cranial nerves No 1,
No 2, etc
NA:
Narcotics Anonymous
neutralizing antibody
nicotinic acid
Nomina Anatomica
noradrenaline
nucleic acid
numerical aperture
nurse's aide
Na:
Avogadro's number
natrium (L) sodium (chemical
symbol for)
^{24}**Na:** radioactive sodium
NAA:
naphthaleneacetic acid
nicotinic acid amide
no apparent abnormalities
NAAP: N-acetyl-4-amino-
phenazone
NAB: novarsenobenzol (neoarsphenamine)
NAC: N-acetyl-L-cysteine
NACOR: National Advisory
Committee on Radiation
NAD:
nicotinamide-adenine
dinucleotide
no acute distress
no appreciable disease
nothing abnormal detected

NADP: nicotinamide-adenine-dinucleotide phosphate

NADPH: NADP (reduced form)

Na$_e$: exchangeable body sodium

NAG: non-agglutinating

NAI: non-accidental injury

NAMH: National Association for Mental Health

NANA: N-acetyl neuraminic acid

NAP:
  nasion pogonion (angle of convexity)
  nucleic acid phosphorus

NAPA: N-acetil-*p*-aminophenol

NAPCA: National Air Pollution Control Administration

NaPG: sodium pregnanediol glucuronide

NAPH: naphthyl

NAPT: National Association for the Prevention of Tuberculosis

NAR: nasal airway resistance

NARAL: National Abortion Rights Action League

NARC:
  narcotic
  narcotics officer
  National Association for Retarded Children

narco:
  narcotics hospital
  narcotics officer
  narcotics treatment center

NARD: National Association of Retail Druggists

NAS:
  nasal
  National Academy of Sciences
  National Association of Sanitarians
  no added salt

NASA: National Aeronautics and Space Administration

NASE: National Association for the Study of Epilepsy

NASEAN: National Association for State Enrolled Assistant Nurses

Nat:
  national
  native
  natural

Natr: *natrium* (L) sodium

NB:
  nota bene (L) note well, take notice
  newborn

Nb: niobium (columbium) (chemical symbol for)

^{95}Nb: radioactive niobium

NBI:
  no bone(y) injury
  non-battle injuries

NBM: nothing by mouth

NBME: National Board of Medical Examiners

NBRT: National Board for Respiratory Therapy

NBS: National Bureau of Standards

NBT: nitroblue tetrazolium

NBTNF: newborn, term, normal, female

NBTNM: newborn, term, normal, male

NBTS: National Blood Transfusion Service

NC:
  nitrocellulose
  no change
  Nurse Corps

nc: nanocurie

NCA:
  National Council on Alcoholism
  neurocirculatory asthenia

NCHS: National Center for Health Statistics

NCHSR: National Center for Health Services Research

NCI:
  naphthalene creosote, iodoform (powder)
  National Cancer Institute

NCIB: National Collection of Industrial Bacteria

NCL: National Chemical Laboratory

NCMH: National Committee for Mental Health

NCMHI: National Clearinghouse for Mental Health Information (HEW)

NCN: National Council of Nurses

NCRND: National Committee for Research in Neurological Diseases

NCRPM: National Committee on Radiation Protection and Measurements

NCSC: National Council of Senior Citizens

NCTC: National Collection of Type Cultures

ND:
natural death
neoplastic disease
neutral density
New Drug
normal delivery
not detected
not determined

N_d: refractive index (symbol for)

Nd:
neodymium (chemical symbol for)
number of dissimilar (matches)

NDA:
National Dental Association
new drug application

NDCR: National Drug Code Directory

NDGA: nordihydro-guairetic acid

NDT: non-destructive testing

NDV: Newcastle disease virus

NE:
National Emergency
nerve excitability (test)
neurological examination
norepinephrine
not enlarged
not examined

Ne: neon (chemical symbol for)

nebul: *nebula* (L) a spray

NEC: not elsewhere classified

NED: normal equivalent deviation

NEEP: negative end expiratory pressure

NEFA: non-esterified fatty acid

neg:
negative (symbol: –)
negro

nem: *Nährungsteinheit Milch* (Ger) nutritional unit milk

NEMA: National Eclectic Medical Association

nema: nematode (threadworm)

neo:
negative expiratory pressure
neoarsphenamine

NEP:
negative expiratory pressure
nephrology

nerv: nervous

NES: not elsewhere specified

n et m: *nocte et mane* (L) night and morning

ne tr s num: *ne tradas sine nummo* (L) do not deliver unless paid

Neurol: neurology

Neuropath: neuropathology(ist)

Neuro-Surg: neurosurgeon(ery)

neut:
neuter
neutral

NF:
National Formulary
negro female
neutral fraction
none found
normal flow

NFC:
National Fertility Center
not favourably considered

NFIP: National Foundation for Infantile Paralysis

NFLPN: National Federation of Licensed Practical Nurses

NFS: National Fertility Study

NFTD: normal full term delivery

NG:
nasogastric
new growth
no good

ng: nanogram (millimicrogram)

NGF: nerve growth factor

NGR: narrow gauze roll

NGU: non-gonococcal urethritis

NH: nursing home

NH_3: ammonia (chemical formula for)

NHI:
National Health Insurance
National Heart Institute

NHLBI: National Heart, Lung, and Blood Institute

NHMRC: National Health and Medical Research Council

NHS:
    National Health Service
    normal human serum
NHSR: National Hospital Service
    Reserve
NI:
    no information
    not found
Ni: nickel (chemical symbol for)
NIA:
    National Institute of Aging
    no information available
NIAB: National Institute of
    Agricultural Botany
NIAID: National Institute of Allergy
    and Infectious Diseases
NIAMD: National Institute of
    Arthritis and Metabolic
    Diseases
Nic: nicotinyl
NICHHD: National Institute of
    Child Health and Human
    Development
NICM: Nuffield Institute of
    Comparative Medicine
NIDR: National Institute of Dental
    Research
NIEHS: National Institute of
    Environmental Health
    Services
NIF: negative inspiratory force
nig: *niger* (L) black
NIGMS: National Institute of
    General Medical Sciences
NIH: National Institutes of Health
    (Bethesda, Md)
NIH 204: an antimalarial drug
NIIP: National Institute of
    Industrial Psychology
NIMH: National Institute of Mental
    Health
NIMR: National Institute for
    Medical Research
NINDB: National Institute of
    Neurological Diseases and
    Blindness (NIH)
NINDS: National Institute of
    Neurological Diseases and
    Stroke
NIOSH: National Institute of
    Occupational Safety and
    Health
NIP: mono-nitroiodophenyl

NIRMP: National Intern and
    Resident Matching Program
NIRNS: National Institute for
    Research in Nuclear Science
NIT: National Intelligence Test
    (psychology)
NK: *Nomenklatur Kommission*
    (Ger) Commission on
    Nomenclature
nl:
    nanolitre
    non licet (L) it is not permitted
    non liquet (L) it is not clear
NLM: National Library of Medicine
NLN: National League for Nursing
NLNE: National League for
    Nursing Education
nlt: not less than
NM:
    negro male
    neuromuscular
    night and morning
    nitrogen mustards
    non-motile (with reference to
    bacteria)
    nuclear medicine
nm:
    nanometre (millimicron)
    nux moschata (L) nutmeg
NMA:
    National Malaria Association
    National Medical Association
NMF: non-migrating fraction (of
    spermatozoa)
NMI: no middle initial
NMN: nicotinamide mono-
    nucleotide
NMR: nuclear magnetic reson-
    ance (spectroscopy
NMRI: Naval Medical Research
    Institute
NMRI448: An insecticide and
    insect repellent
NMSS: National Multiple Sclerosis
    Society
NMT: neuromuscular tension
NMTS: National Milk Testing
    Service
NMU: neuromuscular unit
N:N: the azo group
nn:
    nerves
    nomen novum (L) new name

NND:
 neonatal death
 New and Non-official Drugs
NNEB: National Nursery Examination Board
NNIP: di-nitroiodophenyl
NNMC: National Naval Medical Center
NNN: Novy-Nicolle-McNeal (bacteriological culture medium)
n nov: *nomen novum* (L) new name
NNR: New and Non-official Remedies
NO:
 narcotics officer
 nitric oxide (chemical formula: N_2O)
No: nobelium (chemical symbol)
no:
 number
 numero (L) to the number of
nob: *nobis* (L) to us (as a new species)
noct:
 nocte (L) at night
 nox, noctis (L) light, nocturnal
noct maneq: *nocte maneque* (L) at night and in the morning
nom dub: *nomen dubium* (L) a doubtful name
nom nov: *nomen novum* (L) new name
nom nud: *nomen nudum* (L) a name without designation
non rep: *non repetatur* (L) do not repeat, no refill
NOP: not otherwise provided for
NOPHN: National Organization for Public Health Nursing
NORC: National Opinion Research Center
norleu: norleucine
norm: normal
NOS: not otherwise specified
NOTB: National Ophthalmic Treatment Board
nov: *novum* (L) new
nov n: *novum nomen* (L) new name
NOVS: National Office of Vital Statistics

nov sp: *novum species* (L) new species
NP:
 nasopharynx
 near point
 neuropsychiatry
 not practised
 nucleoplasmic (index)
 nucleoprotein
 nurse practitioner
 nursing procedure
Np: neptunium (chemical symbol)
np: *nomen proprium* (L) proper name (label with)
NPC: near point of convergence
NPD: Niemann-Pick's disease
NPH: neutral protamine Hagedorn (insulin)
NPI: Neuro-psychiatric Institute
NPL: National Physics Laboratory
NPN: nonprotein nitrogen
NPO: *non per os* (L) nothing by mouth
NPRL: Navy Prosthetics Research Laboratory
NPT: normal pressure and temperature
NR:
 do not repeat (in prescriptions)
 neutral red (an indicator)
 non-rebreathing
 no refill (in prescriptions)
 no report
 no response
 normal range
 nutritive ratio
nr: near
NRbc: nucleated red blood cell (mass)
NRC:
 National Research Council
 normal retinal correspondence
NRDL: Naval Radiological Defense Laboratory
NREM: non-rapid eye movement
NRRL: Northern Regional Research Laboratory
NRS: normal rabbit serum
NRSFPS: National Reporting System for Family Planning Services
NS:
 nervous system

neurosurgery, neurosurgeon
normal saline
normal serum

ns:
nanosecond
no sequelae
no specimen
not significant
nylon suture

NDA: Neurological Society of America

nsa:
no salt added
no significant abnormalities

NSAID: non-steroidal anti-inflammatory drug

NSC: non-service connected

NSCC: National Society for Crippled Children

NSD:
no significant defect
no significant deficiency
normal spontaneous delivery

NSDP: National Society of Dental Prosthetists

nsec: nanosecond

NSF: National Science Foundation

NSFTD: normal spontaneous full-term delivery

NSG: neurosecretory granules

nsg: nursing

NSILA: non-suppressible insulin-like activity

NSMA: National Society for Medical Research

Nsn: number of similar negative (matches)

NSNA: National Student Nurse Association

Nsp: number of similar positive (matches)

NSPB: National Society for the Prevention of Blindness

NSR: normal sinus rhythm

NSS: normal saline solution

NSU: non-specific urethritis

NSurg: neurosurgery

NT:
nasotracheal
neotetrazolium (histological stain)
neutralization test
no test

N&T: nose and throat

Nt: niton (chemical symbol for)

NTA:
National Tuberculosis Association
nitrilotriacetic acid
Nursery Training Association

NTG: nitroglycerine

NTIS: National Technical Information Service (formerly CFSTI)

NTP:
normal temperature and pressure
nucleoside triphosphate

NTR: nutrition

nU: nanounit (one billionth or 10^{-9} of a standard unit)

nuc: nucleated

nucl: nucleus

NUG: necrotizing ulcerative gingivitis

NUI: National University of Ireland

NV:
next visit
non-vaccinated
non-venereal
non-veteran
non-volatile

N&V: nausea and vomiting

Nv: naked vision

NVM: non-volatile matter

NW: naked weight

NWB: non-weight-bearing

NWF: National War Formulary

NYAS: New York Academy of Science

NYD: not yet diagnosed

NYHA: New York Heart Association

NYP: not yet published

nyst: nystagmus

O

O:
no special preparation necessary (for test)
occiput

occlusal
octarius (L) pint
oculus (L) eye
ohne Hauch (Ger) symbol
    designating a non-mobile
    type of micro-organism
old
opening of an electric circuit
operator
operon (genetics)
opium
oral(ly)
orange (an indicator colour)
oxygen (chemical symbol for)
without film (bact.)
o-: ortho- (in chemical com-
    pounds)
O_2:
both eyes (symbol for)
oxygen (symbol for the diatomic
    gas)
O_2 sat: oxygen saturation
O_3: ozone (symbol for)
OA:
occiput anterior
old age
osteoarthritis
OAA:
Old Age Assistance
oxaloacetic acid
OAAD: ovarian ascorbic acid
    depletion (test)
OADC: oleic acid, albumin, dex-
    trose, catalase (medium)
OAF: open air factor
O antigens: Somatic antigens
    (those associated with cyto-
    plasm and cell wall of bac-
    teria)
OAP:
Old Age Pension(er)
ophthalmic artery pressure
OAS:
Old Age Security
Organisation of American
    States
OASDHI: Old Age, Survivors, Dis-
    ability and Health Insurance
    (Program)
OASI: Old Age and Survivors
    Insurance
OASP: organic acid soluble
    phosphorus

OB: obstetrics
ob: *obiit* (L) he died; she died
OBE:
Office of Biological Education
Order of the British Empire
OBG: obstetrician-gynaecologist
OB-GYN: obstetrics-gynaecology
obl: oblique
OBS:
obstetrics
organic brain syndrome
Obs:
observer(ed)
obsolete
Obst: obstetrics(tian)
obst: obstruction
OC:
occlusocervical
office call
only child
oral contraceptive
oxygen consumed
O&C: onset and course (of a dis-
    ease)
Occ:
occasionally
occlusion
OccTh: occupational therapy(ist)
Occup: occupation(al)
OCD:
Office of Civil Defence
ovarian cholesterol depletion
    (test)
OCT: ornithine carbonyl trans-
    ferase
Octup: *octuplus* (L) eight-fold
OCV: ordinary conversational
    voice
OD:
Doctor of Optometry
occupational disease
oculus dexter (L) right eye
open drop
optical density
originally derived
out-of-date
outside diameter
overdose
od: *omni die* (L) every day, daily
    once daily
ODA: *occipito-dextra anterior* (L)
    right occipito-anterior
    (position of fetus)

Odont: odontology

odoram: *odoramentum* (L) a perfume

odorat: *odoratus* (L) odorous, smelling, perfuming

ODP: *occipito-dextra posterior* (L) right occipito-posterior (position of fetus)

ODT: *occipitodextra transverse* (L) right occipito-transverse (position of fetus)

OE:
on examination
otitis externa

O&E: observation and examination

OEE: outer enamel epithelium

OEM: open-end marriage

OER: oxygen enhancement ratio

oesoph: oesophagus

OF: occipital-frontal (diameter of head)

O/F: oxidation/fermentation (medium)

Off: official

OG:
Obstetrics-Gynecology
occlusogingival
orange green (stain)

OGTT: oral glucose tolerance test

OH:
hydroxyl radical
occupational health
occupational history
Outpatient Hospital

OHC: outer hair cells

17-OHCS: 17-hydroxy-cortico-steroid

OHD: organic heart disease

OHI: ocular hypertension indicator

OI:
opsonic index
orgasmic impairment
oxygen income or intake

OIH: ovulation-inducing hormone

oint: ointment

OIT: organic integrity test (psychiatry)

OJ: orange juice

OK: correct, approved, all right

OL: *oculus laevus* (L) left eye

Ol: *oleum* (L) oil

OLA: *occipitolaeva anterior* (L) left

occipito-anterior (position of fetus)

Ol oliv: *oleum olivea* (L) olive oil

OLP: *occipitolaeva posterior* (L) left occipito-posterior (position of fetus)

Ol res: oleoresin

OLT: *occipitolaeva transversa* (L) left occipito-transverse (position of fetus)

OM:
occipitomental (diameter of head)
Occupational Medicine
osteomyelitis
otitis media

om: *omni mane* (L) every morning

Ω:
omega (twenty-fourth letter of Greek alphabet
ohm

omn bih: *omni bihora* (L) every two hours

omn hor: *omni hora* (L) every hour

omn 2 hor: *omni secunda hora* (L) every two hours

omn man: *omni mane* (L) every morning

omn noct: *omni nocte* (L) every night

omn quad hor: *omni quadrante hora* (L) every quarter of an hour

OMPA: octamethyl pyrophos-phoramide (an anticholin-esterase

OM&S: Osteopathic Medicine and Surgery

ON: Orthopaedic Nurse

on: *omni nocte* (L) every night

ONC: Orthopaedic Nursing Certificate

OND: Ophthalmic Nursing Diploma

ONP: operating nursing procedure

OOB: out of bed

OOLR: ophthalmology, otology, laryngology, rhinology

OP:
occiput posterior
operative procedure
osmotic pressure

outpatient
overproof
ovine prolactin
op:
operation
Ophthalmic Nurse
opposite
other than psychotic
opus (L) work
O&P: ova and parasites
OPC: Outpatient Clinic
op cit: *opus citatum* (L) in the work cited
OPD:
optical path difference
Outpatient Department
Outpatient Dispensary
OpDent: operative dentistry
opg: opening
OPH: ophthalmology
Oph: ophthalmoscope(ic)
Ophth: ophthalmology(ic)
opp: opposed, opposite
OPS: Out-Patient Service
opt:
optician
optics(ical)
optimum
optional
OPV: oral poliovirus vaccine
OR:
operating room
Orthopaedic Research
O-R: oxidation-reduction
ORANS: Oak Ridge Analytical Systems
Ord: orderly
OREF: Orthopedic Research and Education Foundation
OR enema: oil retention enema
org: organic
organiz: organization(al)
ORIF: open reduction with internal fixation
orig: origin(al)
OrJ: orange juice
ORL: otorhinolaryngology
ORN:
Operating Room Nurse
Orthopaedic Nurse
Orn: ornithine
ORS:
oral surgeon

Orthopaedic Research Society
orthopaedic surgeon(ery)
ORT: operating room technician
Ortho: orthopaedics
OS:
oculus sinister (L) left eye
Osgood-Schlatter's (disease)
osteogenic sarcoma
Os:
bone (L)
mouth (L)
osmium (chemical symbol for)
OSA: Optical Society of America
OSHA: Occupational Safety and Health Act
OSM: osmol
osm: osmotic
OSRD: Office of Scientific Research and Development (USA)
OSS: Office of Strategic Services (US)
OST: Office of Science and Technology
Osteo:
osteomyelitis
osteopath(thy)
OStJ: Officer of the Order of St John of Jerusalem
OSTS: Office of State Technical Services
OSUK: Ophthalmological Society of the United Kingdom
OT:
objective test (psychology)
occupational therapy(ist)
old term
old tuberculin
orotracheal
otology
Ot: otolaryngology(ist)
OTA:
Office of Technology Assessment
orthotoluidine arsenite (test for blood in urine)
OTC:
ornithine transcarbamylase
over-the-counter (with reference to drugs not requiring a prescription)
oxytetracycline
OTD: organ tolerance dose

OTM: orthotolidine manganese sulphate
OTO: otology
Otol: otology(ist)
OTR:
  ovarian tumour registry
  Registered Occupational Therapist
OTReg: Occupational Therapist Registered (Canada)
OU:
  oculi unitas (L) both eyes together
  oculus uterque (L) for each eye
OV:
  office visit
  overventilation (hyperventilation)
ov: *ovum* (L) egg
OVD: occlusal vertical dimension
OW:
  ordinary warfare
  out-of-wedlock
O/W: oil in water (with reference to emulsions)
ox: oxymel (honey, water, and vinegar)
oz: ounce

P

P:
  page
  pain
  parte (L) part
  partial pressure or tension
  Pasteurella
  pater (L) father
  per (L) by
  percentile
  perceptual speed
  percussion
  peyote
  pharmacopoeia
  phenolphthalein (an indicator)
  phosphate
  phosphorus (chemical symbol for)
  pink (an indicator colour)
  plasma
  pole

pondere (L) by weight
poise
population
porcelain
position
positive
posterior
postpartum
premolar
presbyopia
President
pressure
primitive (with reference to haemoglobin)
probability
product
prolactin
proximum (L) near
psychiatry(ist)
pugillus (L) handful
pulse
punctum proximum (L) near point (of vision)
pupil
p:
  page
  papilla (optic)
  pico (prefix)
  pint
  post (L) after
  pupil
π**:** pi (sixteenth letter of the Greek alphabet)
p-: *para-* (in chemical formulas)
P$_1$: first parental generation (in genetics)
P$_2$: second pulmonic heart sound
^{32}P: radioactive phosphorus
P-55: hydroxypregnanedione (a depressant)
PA:
  paralysis agitans
  pernicious anaemia
  phosphoarginine
  photoallergenic (response)
  Physician's Assistant
  platelet adhesiveness
  posteroanterior
  prior to admission
  prolonged action
  proprietary association
  psychoanalyst
  psychogenic aspermia

pulmonary artery
pulpo-axial
P$_A$: partial pressure in arterial blood
Pa:
Pascal
protactinium (chemical symbol for)
P&A: percussion and auscultation
3-PAA: 3 pyridineacetic acid
PAB: *para*-aminobenzoic (acid)
PABA: *para*-aminobenzoic acid
PAC:
parent-adult-child (in transactional analysis)
phenacetin (acetophenetidin), aspirin, caffeine
premature atrial contraction
PAD: phenacetin, aspirin, desoxyephedrine
pae: *partes aequales* (L) in equal parts
paed: paediatrics
PAF: pulmonary arteriovenous fistula
PA&F: percussion, auscultation, and fremitus
PAGE: polyacrylamide gel electrophoresis
PAH: *para*-aminohippuric acid (used in kidney function tests)
PAHO: Pan-American Health Organization
PAL:
Pathology Laboratory (test)
posterior axillary line
palp: palpable
palpi: palpitation
PAM:
crystalline penicillin G in 2% aluminium monostearate
melphalan/phenylalanine mustard
pam: pamphlet
PAN: peroxyacetyl nitrate
PAP: primary atypical pneumonia
Pap: Papanicolaou (diagnosis, smear, stain, or test)
pap: papilla, papillae
PAPS: adenosine-3′ phosphate-5′- sulphonatophosphate

PAR: postanaesthetic recovery (room)
par: parafine
Para: Formula designating: P—number of pregnancies; a—number of abortions or miscarriages; ra— number of living children (e.g. Para 4-2-1 means 4 pregnancies, 2 abortions or miscarriages, 1 living child)
Para I: unipara (having borne one child)
Para II: bipara (having borne two children)
Para III: tripara (having borne three children)
par aff: *pars affecta* (L) to the part affected
Parapsych: parapsychology
parasym div: parasympathetic division (of autonomic nervous system)
parent: parenteral(ly)
parox: paroxysmal
part: *partim* (L) part
part aeq: *partes aequales* (L) in equal parts
part vic: *partibus vicibus* (L) in divided doses
PARU: postanaesthetic recovery unit
parv: *parvus* (L) small
PAS:
p-aminosalicylic acid
periodic-acid-Schiff (stain)
Professional Activities Study (Commission on Professional and Hospital Activities)
PASA: *para*-aminosalicylic acid (used in treatment of tuberculosis)
P'ase: alkaline phosphatase
pass: passive
Past: *Pasteurella*
PAT:
paroxysmal atrial tachycardia
preganancy at term
pat: patent(ed)
PATE: Psychodynamic and Therapeutic Education
Path:
pathogenic

pathological
pathology(ist)
pat med: patent medicine
PB:
British Pharmacopeia
phenobarbitone(al)
phonetically balanced (with
reference to word lists)
pressure breathing
Pb:
plumbum (L) lead (chemical
symbol for)
presbyopia
PBA: Pressure Breathing Assister
PBB: polybromated biphenyls
PBC: point of basal convergence
PBE: *Persucht Bacillen-Emulsion*
(Ger) (a form of tuberculin)
PBG: porphobilinogen
PBI:
phenformin (oral hypoglycaemic
agent)
protein-bound iodine
PBK: phosphorylase b kinase
PBS: phosphate buffered saline
PBW: posterior bite wing
(dentistry)
PBZ:
phenylbutazone
pyribenzamine
PC:
packed cells
parent cells
phosphatidylcholine (lecithin)
phosphocreatine
Physicians Corporation
platelet concentrate
pneumotaxic centre
pondus civile (L) avoirdupois
weight
postcoital
praecordium
present complaint
pubococcygeus (muscle)
pulmonary capillary
pc:
per cent
picocurie
post cibos (L) after meals
post cibum (L) after food
PCA: passive cutaneous anaphylaxis
PCB: polychlorinated biphenyls

PcB: near point of convergence to
the intercentral base line
PCC:
phaeochromocytoma
phosphate carrier compound
Poison Control Center
PCc: periscopic concave
PCD: polycystic disease
PCF:
pharyngoconjunctival fever
prothrombin conversion factor
PCG: phonocardiogram
PCH: paroxysmal cold haemo-
globinuria
pCi: picocurie
PCIC: Poison Control Information
Center
PCL: persistent corpus luteum
PCM: protein-calorie malnutrition
PCMO: Principal Colonial Medical
Officer
PCN: pregnenolone carbonitril
PCNV: Provisional Committee on
Nomenclature of Viruses
PCO: patient complains of
PCOB: Permanent Central Opium
Board (Geneva)
PCo$_2$: carbon dioxide pressure or
tension (symbol for)
PCP: pentachlorophenol
PCPA: *p*-chlorophenylalanine
pcpn: precipitation
pcpt: perception
pcs: preconscious
PCT:
plasmacrit test (syphilis)
porphyria cutanea tarda
proximal convoluted tubule (of a
nephron)
pct: per cent
PCV:
packed cell volume
polycythaemia vera
PCx: periscopic convex
PD:
Doctor of Pharmacy
Dublin Pharmacopoeia
interpupillary distance
paediatrics
paralysing dose
parkinsonism dementia
Parkinson's disease
pars distalis (pituitary)

phenyldichlorarsine (a war gas)
phosphate dextrose (media)
potential difference
pressor dose
psychotic depression
Pd: palladium (chemical symbol for)
pd:
papilla diameter
per diem (L) by the day
prism diopter
pupillary distance
PDA:
paediatric allergy
patent ductus arteriosus
PDB: paradichlorobenzene
PDC:
paediatrics-cardiology
penta-decylcatechol
preliminary diagnostic clinic
private diagnostic clinic
PDE: paroxysmal dyspnoea on exertion
PDGA: pteroyldiglutamic acid
PDH: past dental history
P-diol: pregnanediol
PDQ: at once; immediately
PDR:
paediatrics-radiology
Physicians' Desk Reference
pdr: powder
PE:
Edinburgh Pharmacopoeia
pharyngoesophageal
phosphatidyl ethanolamine
physical examination
potential energy
powdered extract
probable error
pulmonary embolism
Pe: pressure on expiration
PEA: phenethyl_alcohol (blood agar)
PED: paediatrics
PEd: physical education
PEDG: phenformin (SEE *PBI*)
PEEP: positive end expiratory pressure
PEF: peak expiratory flow
PEG:
pneumoencephalogram(phy)
polyethylene glycol
PEI: phosphorus excretion index

penic: pencillin
penic cam: *penicillum camelinum* (L) camel's-hair brush
Pent: pentothal
PEP:
phosphoenolpyruvate
polyoestradiol phosphate
PEPR: precision encoder and pattern recognizer
per:
by; through
period
periodic
person
perf: perforation(ed)
periap: periapical
PERLA: pupils equal, react to light and accommodation
perm: permanent
per op emet: *peracta operatione emetici* (L) when the action of the emetic is over
perp: perpendicular
PERRLA: pupils equal, round, react to light and accommodation
pers: personal
pert: pertussis (whooping cough)
PET: pre-eclamptic toxaemia
PETN: pentaerythrityl tetranitrate (a coronary dilator)
petr: petroleum
PF:
peak flow
permeability factor
plantar flexion
platelet factor
pulmonary factor
Pf: *Pfeifferella*
PFA: *para*-fluorophenylalanine
PFC: plaque-forming cells
PFD: primary flash distillate
PFK: phosphofructokinase
PFO: patent foramen ovale
PFR: peak flow rate (reading)
PFT: pulmonary function test
PFU:
plaque-forming unit
pock-forming units
PFV: physiological full value
PG:
glycerate-3-phosphate
paregoric

Pharmacopoeia Germanica
postgraduate
pregnanedioi glucuronide
prostaglandin
Pg: pregnant
pg: picogram
6-PG: 6-phosphogluconate
PGA:
  prostaglandin A
  pteroylglutamic acid (folic acid)
PGB: prostaglandin B
PGDF; Pilot Guide Dog Foundation
PGE: prostaglandin E
PGF: prostaglandin F
PGH: pituitary growth hormone
PGM: phosphoglucomutase
PGR: psychogalvanic response
PGU: postgonococcal urethritis
PGUT: phosphogalactose-uridyl transferase
PH:
  past history
  previous history
  public health
Ph:
  pharmacopoeia
  phenyl
  phosphate
pH: Symbol for expression of hydrogen ion concentration
ph: phial
PHA:
  passive haemagglutination
  phytohaemagglutinin
phaeo: phaeochromocytoma
phar(m):
  pharmacopoeia
  pharmacy(ceutical)
PharB: *Pharmaciae Baccalaureus* (L) Bachelor of Pharmacy
PharC: Pharmaceutical Chemist
PharD: *Pharmaciae Doctor* (L) Doctor of Pharmacy
PharG: Graduate in Pharmacy
PharM: *Pharmaciae Magister* (L) Master of Pharmacy
PhB:
  Bachelor of Philosophy
  British Pharmacopoeia
PHC: posthospital care
PhC: Pharmaceutical Chemist
Ph¹c: Philadelphia chromosome

PhD: Doctor of Philosophy
PHE: post-heparin esterase
Phe: phenylalanine
Pheo: phaeochromocytoma
PhG:
  Graduate in Pharmacy
  Pharmacopoeia Germanica
Phgly: phenylglycine
PHI: phosphohexose isomerase
PhI: Pharmacopoeia Internationalis
phial: *phiala* (L) bottle
PHK cells: postmortem human kidney cells
PHLA: post-heparin lipolytic activity
PHLS: Public Health Laboratory Service
PHN: Public Health Nursing
phos:
  phosphate
  phosphorus
PHP:
  post-heparin phospholipase
  prepaid health plan
  pseudohypoparathyroidism
PHS: Public Health Service
PHTS: Psychiatric Home Treatment Service
PhyS: physiological saline
Phys: physician
phys: physical
phys dis: physical disability
PhysEd: physical education
physio: physiotherapy(ist)
Physiol: physiology(ical)
PhysMed: physical medicine
PhysTher: physical therapy
PI:
  patient's interests
  Pharmacopeia Internationalis
  present illness
  primary infarction
  proactive inhibition (psychology)
  protamine insulin
  Protocol Internationale (International Protocol)
  pulmonary incompetence
Pi: pressure of inspiration
PIC:
  Population Investigation Committee
  postinflammatory corticoid

PICU: Pulmonary Intensive Care Unit

PID:
pelvic inflammatory disease
photoionization detector
prolapsed intervertebral disc

PIE: pulmonary infiltration associated with eosinophilia

PIF:
prolactin release inhibiting factor
proliferation inhibiting factor

PIFR: peak inspiratory flow rate

pil: *pilula* (L) pill

ping: *pinguis* (L) fat, grease

PIP: proximal interphalangeal (joint)

PIRP: Provisional International Reference Preparation

PIS: Provisional International Standard

PITR: plasma iron turnover rate

PIV: parainfluenza virus

PK:
Prausnitz-Küstner (reaction)
psychokinesis
pyruvate kinase

pK: dissociation constant

pKa: negative log of dissociation constant

PKU: phenylketonuria

PL:
perception of light
phospholipid
placental lactogen
plastic surgeon(ery)
pulpolingual

pl:
place
plate
plural

PLA: pulpolinguoaxial

PLa: pulpolabial

plant-flex: plantar flexion

PLD: potentially lethal damage

P-LGV: psittacosis-lymphogranuloma venereum

PLP: pyridoxal phosphate

PLT: psitticosis-lymphogranuloma-trachoma

plumb: *plumbum* (L) lead

plx: plexus

PM:
petit mal
physical medicine
post meridiem (L) after noon
post mortem (L) after death
premolar
presystolic murmur
preventative medicine
prostatic massage
pulpomesial

Pm: promethium (chemical symbol for) (formerly illinium)

PMA:
papillary, marginal, attached (with reference to gingivae)
Pharmaceutical Manufacturers Association
Primary Mental Abilities (test)
progressive muscular atrophy
pyridylmercuric acetate

PMB:
polychrome methylene blue
polymorphonuclear basophils
post-menopausal bleeding

PMC: phenylmercuric chloride

PMD: progressive muscular dystrophy

PMd: private physician

PME: polymorphonuclear eosinophils

PMF: progressive massive fibrosis

PMH: past medical history

PMI:
past (previous) medical illness
point of maximal impulse (of heart on chest wall)
point of maximum intensity

PML:
polymorphonuclear leucocytes
progressive multifocal leucoencephalopathy

PMN: polymorphonuclear neutrophilic (leucocytes)

PMNR: periadenitis mucosa necrotica recurrens

PMO: Principal Medical Officer

PMP:
persistent mentoposterior (position of fetus)
previous menstrual period

PMR: protein magnetic resonance

PM&R: physical medicine and rehabilitation

PMRAFNS: Princess Mary's Royal Air Force Nursing Service

PMRS: Physical Medicine and Rehabilitation Service

PMS:
chorionic gonadotrophin in pregnant mare's serum
phenasinemethosulphate
poor miserable soul
post-menopausal syndrome
pregnant mare's serum

PMSG: pregnant mare's serum gonadotrophin

PMT: premenstrual tension

PN:
percussion note
periarteritis nodosa
peripheral nerve
postnatal
Practical Nurse
psychiatry-neurology
psycho-neurologist
psychoneurotic individual

Pn: pneumonia

P&N: psychiatry and neurology

PNA:
Nomina Anatomica (Paris) (with reference to anatomical nomenclature)
pentosenucleic acid

PNAvQ: positive-negative ambivalent quotient (psychology)

PNBT: *para*-nitroblue tetrazoleum

PNC: penicillin

PND:
paroxysmal nocturnal dyspnoea
postnasal drip or drainage

PNed: *Nederlandsche Pharmacopee* (Dutch pharmacopoeia)

PNF: proprioceptive neuromuscular facilitation

PNH: paroxysmal nocturnal haemoglobinuria

PNI:
peripheral nerve injury
postnatal infection

PNMT: phenylethanolamine-N-methyl transferase

PNO: Principal Nursing Officer

P-NP: *p*-nitrophenol

PNPR: positive-negative pressure respiration

P-NPS: *p*-nitrophenylsulphate

PNS:
parasympathetic nervous system
peripheral nervous system

PNU: protein nitrogen unit

Pnx: pneumothorax

PO:
period of onset
phone order
postoperative

Po: polonium (chemical symbol for)

po: *per os* (L) by mouth

PO_2: oxygen tension or pressure

PO_4: phosphate

POA: primary optic atrophy

POB: penicillin, oil beeswax

pocill: *pocillum* (L) a small cup

pocul: *poculum* (L) cup

PODx: preoperative diagnosis

POF: pyruvate oxidation factor

PofE: portal of entry

pOH: Symbol used in expressing hydroxyl (OH) concentration or alkalinity of a solution

pois: poison

pol: polish (dentistry)

polio: poliomyelitis

Poly: polymorphonuclear leucocyte or neutrophil granulocyte

PolyIC: polyisosinic-polycytidylic (acid)

POMR: problem oriented medical record

pond: *pondere* (L) by weight

POP:
persistent occipitoposterior (position of fetus)
plasma osmotic pressure
plaster of paris

POp: postoperative

Pop:
popliteal
population

pop: popular

pos:
position
positive

POSM: patient-operated selector mechanism

POSS: proximal over-shoulder strap
post:
  posterior
  post mortem (autopsy)
postgangl: postganglionic
post-op: postoperative
pot:
  potassium
  potential
  potion
potass: potassium
POU: placenta, ovary, uterus
powd: powder
PP:
  partial pressure
  posterior pituitary
  postpartum
  postprandial
  private patient
  private practice
  pulse pressure
  pyrophosphate
pp: *punctum proximum* (L) near point of accommodation (in respect to vision)
ppa: *phiala prius agitate* (L) the bottle having first been shaken
pp&a: palpation, percussion, and auscultation
PPB: positive pressure breathing
ppb: parts per billion
PPC: progressive patient care
PPCA: plasma prothrombin conversion accelerator
PPCF: plasma prothrombin conversion factor
PPD:
  progressive perceptive deafness
  purified protein derivative (tuberculin)
PPD-S: purified protein derivative-standard
PPF: pellagra preventive factor (niacinamide)
PPFA: Planned Parenthood Federation of America
ppg: picopicogram
PPH: post-partum haemorrhage
PPHP: pseudo-pseudohypo-parathyroidism

PPLO: pleuropneumonia-like organisms
ppm: parts per million
PPO: pleuropneumonia organisms
PPP: platelet-poor plasma
PPS: postpartum sterilization
PPT: partial prothrombin time
ppt:
  precipitate
  prepared
pptd: precipitated
PPTL: postpartum tubal ligation
pptn: precipitation
PQ: permeability quotient
PR:
  Panama red (var. of marijuana)
  patient relations
  percentile rank
  peripheral resistance
  phenol red (an indicator)
  pityriasis rosea
  pregnancy rate
  pressoreceptor
  proctologist
  progressive resistance
  prosthetic-group removing (enzyme)
  prosthion
  pulse rate
Pr:
  praseodymium (chemical symbol for)
  presbyopia
  prism
  prolactin
  propyl (normal)
pr:
  pair
  per rectum
  punctum remotum (L) far point of accommodation (in respect to vision)
PRA: plasma renin activity
prac: practice
pract: practical
prand: *prandium* (L) dinner
PRAS: prereduced anaerobically sterilized (media)
p rat aetat: *pro ratione aetatis* (L) in proportion to age
PRB: Prosthetics Research Board

PRC: plasma renin concentration

PRD: partial reaction of degeneration

PRE: progressive resistive exercise

Pre: preliminary

p rec: per rectum

precip: precipitate(ion)

pred: predicted

prefd: preferred

preg: pregnant

pregn: pregnant

pregang: preganglionic

prelim: preliminary

prelim diag: preliminary diagnosis

prem:
premature
premature infant

pre-op: preoperative

prep: prepare(ation)

prepd: prepared

prepn: preparation

preserv: preserve(ation)

press: pressure

prev:
prevent(ion)(ative)
previous

pre-voc: pre-vocational

PRF: prolactin-releasing factor

PRH: prolactin-releasing hormone

PRIH: prolactin-release inhibiting hormone

prin: principal

priv: private

PRL: prolactin

prn: *pro re nata* (L) as required, whenever necessary

Pro:
proline
prophylactic
prothrombin

prob:
probability
probable(y)
problem

proc:
procedure
proceeding
process

Procs: proceedings

Proct: proctology(ist)

prod: product

Prof: professor

prof: profession(al)

prog:
prognosis
program

progn: prognosis

progr: progress

proj: project

prolong: *prolongatus* (L) prolonged

PROM: preventative rupture of membranes

pron: pronation

proph: prophylactic

pro rect: *pro recto* (L) by rectum

pros: prostate

prosth: prosthesis

Prot: Protestant

prot: protein

pro-time: prothrombin time

PROTO: protoporphyrin

prox: proximal

prox luc: *proxima luce* (L) the day before

PRP: platelet-rich plasma

PRPP: phosphoribosyl pyrophosphate

PRT: phosphoribosyl transferase

PRU: peripheral resistance unit

PS:
chloropicrin (a war gas)
paradoxical sleep
patient's serum
phosphatidyl serine
photosystems
physical status
plastic surgery
point of symmetry
postscriptum
pulmonary stenosis
serum from a pregnant woman

Ps:
prescription (with reference to drugs requiring a prescription)
Pseudomonas

P&S:
paracentesis and suction (with reference to thoracic surgery)
Physicians and Surgeons

PSAn: psychoanalyst (lysis)(ic)(ical)

PSE: point of subjective equality (psychology)

PSI:
  posterior sagittal index
  Problem Solving Information (apparatus)
psi: pounds per square inch
psia: pounds per square inch absolute
psig: pounds per square inch gauge
PSIL: preferred-frequency speech interference level
PSL sol: potassium, sodium chloride, sodium lactate solution
PSMA: progressive spinal muscular atrophy
P sol: partly soluble
PSP: phenolsulphonphthalein (phenol red)
psp: postsynaptic potential
PSRO: Professional Standards Review Organization
PSS:
  physiological saline solution
  progressive systemic sclerosis
PST: penicillin, streptomycin and tetracycline
PSurg: plastic surgery
PSW: Psychiatric Social Worker
Psy: psychiatry
psych: psychology
psychiat: psychiatry(ic)
psychoan: psychoanalysis
psychol: psychology
psychopathol: psychopatho- logy(ical)
psychophys: psychophysics
psychophysiol: psychophysio- logy
psychother: psychotherapy
psy-path: psychopath(ic)
psy-som: psychosomatic
PT:
  parathyroid
  patient
  phototoxity
  physical therapy
  physical training
  physiotherapy
  propylthiouracil
  prothrombin time
  pulmonary tuberculosis
Pt: platinum (chemical symbol for)

pt:
  part
  patient
  perstetur (L) let it be continued
  pint
  point
PTA:
  plasma thromboplastin ante- cedent (Factor XI)
  post-traumatic amnesia
  prior to admission
PTAP: purified toxoid (diphtheria) precipitated by aluminium phosphate
PTB:
  patellar tendon bearing
  prior to birth
PTC:
  phenylthiocarbamide
  plasma thromboplastin com- ponent (Factor IX, Christmas factor)
PTD: permanent total disability
PTE: parathyroid extract
PTEN: pentaerythritol tetranitrate
PTF: plasma thromboplastin factor (Factor X)
PTH:
  parathormone (parathyroid hormone)
  phenylthiohydantoin
  post-transfusion hepatitis
PTM: phenyltrimethylammonium
PTO: *Perlsucht-tuberculin original* (Ger)
PTR: *Perlsucht-tuberculin rest* (Ger)
PTT: partial thromboplastin time
PTU: propylthiouracil (an anti- thyroid drug)
PTx: parathyroidectomy
PTZ: pentylenetetrazol
PU:
  pass urine
  peptic ulcer
  per urethram
  pregnancy urine
Pu:
  plutonium (chemical symbol for)
  purple (an indicator colour)
pub:
  public
  publisher

PuD: pulmonary disease
PUFA: polyunsaturated fatty acid
PUH: pregnancy urine hormone
pulm:
pulmentum (L) gruel
pulmonary
pulv: *pulvis* (L) powder
pulv gros: *pulvis grossus* (L) a coarse powder
pulv subtil: *pulvis subtilis* (L) a smooth powder
pulv tenu: *pulvis tenuis* (L) an extremely fine powder
PUO: pyrexia of unknown origin
purg: *purgativus* (L) cathartic, purgative
PV:
paraventricular (nucleus)
per vaginam
plasma volume
polycythaemia vera
portal vein
pressure/volume
PVA: polyvinyl alcohol (fixative)
PVC:
polyvinylchloride
premature ventricular contraction
PVD:
peripheral vascular disease
pulmonary vascular disease
P-VL: Panton-Valentine leucocidin
PVM: pneumonia virus of mice
PVP: polyvinylpyrrolidone
PVT:
pressure, volume, temperature
private patient
pvt: private
PWC: physical working capacity
PWP: pulmonary wedge pressure
PX: physical examination
Px:
past history
pneumothorax
prognosis
Py: phosphopyridoxal
PYA: psychoanalysis
PYC: proteose-yeast, castione (medium)
PyC: pyogenic culture
PYGM: peptone-yeast glucose maltose (agar/broth)

PYM: psychosomatic medicine
Pyr: pyridine
PyrP: pyridoxyl (pyridoxamine) phosphate
PZ: pancreozymin
PZA: pyrazinamide (pyrazinoic acid amide)
PZI: protamine zinc insulin

Q

Q:
electric quantity
quantity
quartile
query or Queensland (fever)
quinacrine (fluorescent method)
quotient
volume of blood
Q_1, Q_2, Q_3: first or lowest quartile, second quartile, third quartile
q: *quaque* (L) each, every
QAC: quaternary ammonium compound
qam: every morning
QAP:
quality assurance program
quinine, atebrin, plasmoquine (treatment)
QARANC: Queen Alexandra's Royal Army Nursing Corps
QARNNS: Queen Alexandra's Royal Naval Nursing Service
QCH: Queen Charlotte's Hospital
QCIM: Quarterly Cumulative Index Medicus
qd: *quaque die* (L) every day
QEONS: Queen Elizabeth's Overseas Nursery Service
QEW: quick early warning (test)
Q fract: quick fraction (with reference to membrane potentials)
qh: *quaque hora* (L) every hour
q2h: *quaque secunda hora* (L) every two hours
q3h: *quaque tertia hora* (L) every three hours
QHNS: Queen's Honorary Nursing Sister
QHP: Honorary Physician to the Queen

QHS: Honorary Surgeon to the Queen

qid: *quater in die* (L) four times a day

QIDN: Queen's Institute of District Nursing

ql: *quantum libet* (L) as much as is desired, as much as you please

qm: *quaque mane* (L) every morning

qn: *quaque nocte* (L) once every night

QNS:
 quantity not sufficient
 Queen's Nursing Sister (of QIDN)

QO₂: oxygen quotient

qod: every other day

QP: quanti-Pirquet (reaction)

qp: *quantum placeat* (L) as much as you please

qpm: every night

qq: *quaque: quoque* (L) each, every, also

qqh: *quaque quarta hora* (L) every four hours

qq hor: *quaque hora* (L) every hour

QR:
 quantum rectum (L) quantity is correct
 quinaldine red

QRS: segment of electro-cardiograph

QRZ: *Quaddel Reaktion Zeit* (Ger) weal reaction time

qs:
 quantum satis (L) sufficient quantity
 quantum sufficit (L) as much as will suffice

q suff: *quantum sufficit* (L) as much as will suffice

QT: Quick's test (for pregnancy or for prothrombin)

qt: quart

quadrupl: *quadruplicato* (L) four times as much

qual: quality(tative)

qual anal: qualitative analysis

quant: quantity(tative)

quant anal: quantitative analysis

quar: quarterly

quat: *quattuor* (L) four

QUI: Queen's University of Ireland

quinq: *quinque* (L) five

quint: *quintus* (L) fifth

quor: *quorum* (L) of which

quot: *quoties* (L) as often as necessary

quotid: *quotidie* (L) daily

qv:
 quantum vis (L) as much as you wish
 quod vide (L) which see

R

R:
 any alkyl group of an alkane
 Bernken's unit (of roentgen-ray exposure)
 organic radical (in chemical formulas)
 race
 racemic
 radioactive mineral
 radiology(ist)
 Rankin (temperature scale)
 reading
 Réaumur (temperature scale)
 rectal
 red (an indicator colour)
 registered trademark
 regulator (gene)
 Reiz (Ger) stimulus
 remotum (L) far
 repressor
 resazurin
 resistance
 resistant (with reference to disease)
 respiration
 response
 rest (in cell cycle)
 reverse Giemsa method
 review
 Rickettsia
 right
 right eye
 roentgen
 roentgenology(ist)

rough (with reference to bacterial colonies)

In formulas of amino acids, denotes characteristic side chain

Symbol for a gas constant (8.315 joules)

R:
recipe (L) take
treatment

R factor: resistance factor (bacteriology)

+**R:** Rinne's test positive (test for hearing) (symbol for)

−**R:** Rinne's test negative (test for hearing) (symbol for)

RA:
radioactive
repeat action
residual air
rheumatoid arthritis
right angle(ulation) (orthopaedics)
right arm
right atrium
rignt auricle

Ra: radium (chemical symbol for)

rac: racemic

Rad: radiotherapy(ist)

rad:
radiation absorbed dose
radical
radius
radix (L) root

RADA:
right acromio-dorso-anterior (position of fetus)
rosin amine D acetate

RADC: Royal Army Dental Corps

Radiol: Radiology(ist)

RADP: right acromio-dorso-posterior (position of fetus)

RAFMS: Royal Air Force Medical Services

RAIU: radioactive iodine uptake

RAM: random access memory

RAMC: Royal Army Medical Corps

rar: right arm reclining or recumbent

RAS: reticular activating system

ras: *rasurae* (L) scrapings or filings

RAST: radio-allergosorbent test

RAT: repeat action tablet

RAV: Roux associated virus

RAVC: Royal Army Veterinary Corps

Rb: rubidium (chemical symbol for)

RBBsB: right bundle-branch system block

RBC:
red blood cell count
red blood corpuscle (cell)

RBD: right border of dullness(of heart to percussion)

RBE: relative biological effectiveness (of radiation)

RBF: renal blood flow

Rb Imp: rubber base impression (dentistry)

RBNA: Royal British Nurses' Association

RC:
red cell (corpuscle)
Red Cross
respiration ceases
Respiratory Care
respiratory centre
retention catheter
Roman Catholic
root canal

Rc: response, conditioned

RCA: red cell agglutination

RCAF: Royal Canadian Air Force

RCAMP: Royal Canadian Army Medical Corps

RCC: Radio-Chemical Centre

RCD: relative cardiac dullness

RCF: relative centrifugal force

RCM:
reinforced clostridial medium
right costal margin
Royal College of Midwives

Rcn: Royal College of Nursing

RCO: aliphatic acyl radical

RCOG: Royal College of Obstetricians and Gynaecologists

RCP: Royal College of Physicians

RCS:
reticulum cell sarcoma
Royal College of Surgeons

RCSE: Royal College of Surgeons, Edinburgh

RCSI: Royal College of Surgeons, Ireland

RCT: Rorschach Content Test

RCU: Respiratory Care Unit
RCVS: Royal College of
   Veterinary Surgeons
RD:
   reaction of degeneration
   registered dietitian
   retinal detachment
   rubber dam
Rd: reading
rd: rutherford (a unit of
   radioactivity)
R&D: research and development
RDA:
   recommended daily allowance
   right dorso-anterior (position of
   fetus)
RdA: reading age
RDE: receptor destroying enzyme
RDH: Registered Dental Hygienist
RDP: right dorsoposterior
   (position of fetus)
RdQ: reading quotient
RDS: respiratory distress
   syndrome
RE:
   radium emanation
   rectal examination
   resting energy
   reticuloendothelium
   right eye
Re: rhenium (chemical symbol for)
readm: readmission
rec:
   recens (L) fresh
   record
   recreation
   recurrent
RECG: radioelectrocardiography
Recip: recipient
Recomm: recommendation
recond: recondition(ing)
reconstr: reconstruction
recryst: recrystallize
rect:
   rectificatus (L) rectified
   rectum
   rectus (muscle)
recur: recurrent(ence)
redig in pulv: *redigatur in pul-*
   verem (L) let it be reduced to
   powder
red in pulv: *reductus in pulverem*
   (L) reduced to a powder

redox: reduction oxidation
REF: renal erythropoietic factor
ref: refer(ence)
ref doc: referring doctor
refl: reflex
ref phys: referring physician
REG:
   Radiation Exposure Guide
   radioencephalogram (graph)
Reg: registered
reg:
   regarding
   region
   regular
regen: regenerate(ion)
reg umb: umbilical region
rehabil: rehabilitation
REL: rate of energy loss
rel:
   related
   relative
reliq: *reliquus* (L) remainder
REM:
   rapid eye movement (sleep)
   roentgen equivalent man
rem: roentgen equivalent man
REMAB: radiation equivalent
   manikin absorption
REMCAL: radiation equivalent
   manikin calibration
ren: *renovetur* (L) renew
ren sem: *renovetum seml* (L) shall
   be renewed only once
REP:
   retrograde pyelogram
   roentgen equivalent physical
rep:
   repetatur (L) let it be repeated
   report
rept:
   repeat
   report
rER: rough endoplasmic reticulum
RES: reticuloendothelial system
Res:
   research
   reserve
   resident(ence)
resist: resistance
resp:
   respiratory(ion)
   responsible
resus: resuscitation

ret: retired
retard: retarded (delayed)
retic count: reticulocyte count
retics: reticulocytes
rev:
  reverse
  review
  revolution
Rev of Sym: review of symptoms
RF:
  Reitland-Franklin (unit)
  relative flow (rate)
  releasing factor
  replicative form
  resistance factor
  respiratory failure
  rheumatic fever
  rheumatoid factor
rf: radio frequency
R_F: rate of flow (chromatography)
RFA: right frontoanterior (position of fetus)
RFC: rosette-forming cells
RFL: right frontolateral (position of fetus)
RFLS: rheumatoid factor-like substance
RFN: Registered Fever Nurse
RFP: right frontoposterior (position of fetus)
RFPS (Glasgow): Royal Faculty of Physicians and Surgeons of Glasgow
RFR: refraction
RFT: right frontotransverse (position of fetus)
RGE: relative gas expansion
RGN: Registered General Nurse
RH:
  radiant heat
  relative humidity
  releasing hormone
  right hand
  right hyperphoria
Rh:
  Rhesus (with reference to blood factors)
  Rhipicephalus
  rhodium (chemical symbol for)
^{106}**Rh:** radioactive rhodium
Rh−: Rhesus negative
Rh+: Rhesus positive
rh: *rhonchi* (L) rales

RHA: Regional Health Authority
RHB: Regional Hospital Board
RHC:
  resin haemoperfusion column
  respirations have ceased
  right hypochondrium
RHCSA: Regional Hospitals Consultants' and Specialists' Association
RHD:
  relative hepatic dullness
  rheumatic heart disease
rheu fev: rheumatic fever
rheu ht dis: rheumatic heart disease
rheum: rheumatic(ism)
RHF: right heart failure
Rhin: rhinology(ist)
Rhiz: *Rhizobium*
RHS: right hand side
RI:
  radiation intensity
  Recovery, Incorporated
  refractive index
  release-inhibiting
  replicative intermediate
  respiratory illness
  retroactive inhibition (psychology)
RIA: radio-immunoassay
RIA-DA: radio-immunoassay double antibody (test)
RIC: Royal Institute of Chemistry
RICM: right intercostal margin
RID: reversible intravas device
RIF: right iliac fossa
RIFC: rat intrinsic factor concentrate
RIGH: rabies immune globulin, human
RIH: right inguinal hernia
RIHSA: radioactive iodinated human serum albumin
RIMR: Rockefeller Institute for Medical Research
RIPH: Royal Institute of Public Health
RIPHH: Royal Institute of Public Health and Hygiene
RIRB: radioiodinated rose bengal
RISA: radioactive iodinated serum albumin

RIT: radio-iodinated triolein

RKY: roentgen kymography

RL:
coarse rales (with reference to auscultation of chest)
reduction level (the reciprocal of respiratory quotient)
right lower
Ringer lactate
stimulus (*Reiz*) limen

RL$_3$: many coarse rales

Rl: medium rales

Rl$_2$: moderate number of medium rales

rl: fine rales

rl$_1$: few fine rales

RLBCD: right lower border of cardiac dullness

RLC: residual lung capacity

RLD:
related living donor
ruptured lumbar disc

RLE: right lower extremity

RLF:
retrolental fibroplasia
right lateral femoral (site of injection)

RLL: right lower lobe (of lung)

RLMD: rat liver mitochondria (and submitochondrial particles derived by) digitonin (treatment)

RLQ: right lower quadrant (of abdomen)

RLR muscle: right lateral rectus muscle (of eye)

RLS: A person who stammers having difficulty in enuciating R, L, and S

RM:
radical mastectomy
range of movement (motion)
respiratory movement

RMA: right mentoanterior (position of fetus)

RMD: retromanubrial dullness

RMK: rhesus monkey kidney

RML:
right mediolateral (episiotomy)
right middle lobe (of lungs)

RMM: read mostly memory

RMN: Registered Mental Nurse (England and Wales)

RMO:
Regional Medical Officer
Resident Medical Officer

RMP:
Regional Medical Program
right mentoposterior (position of fetus)

RMPA: Royal Medico-Psychological Association

RMR muscle: right medial rectus muscle (of eye)

RMS: square root of mean square

RMSF: Rocky Mountain spotted fever

RMT: right mentotransverse (position of fetus)

RMV: respiratory minute volume

RN:
Registered Nurse
Royal Navy

Rn: radon (chemical symbol for)

RNA:
Registered Nurse Anesthetist
ribonucleic acid
rough, non-capsulated, avirulent (with reference to bacteria)

RNase: ribonuclease

RNIB: Royal National Institute for the Blind

RNID: Royal National Institute for the Deaf

RNMD: Registered Nurse for Mental Defectives

RNMS: Registered Nurse for Mentally Subnormal

Rnt: roentgenology(ist)

RO: routine order

R/O: rule out

ROA: right occipitoanterior (position of fetus)

Roent: roentgenology(ist)

ROL: right occipitolateral (position of fetus)

ROM:
range of movement (motion)
read only memory

RNP: ribonucleoprotein

Rom: Romberg

ROP: right occipitoposterior (position of fetus)

Ror: Rorschach (test)

ROS: review of systems

ROT:
 remedial occupational therapy
 right occipitotransverse
  (position of fetus)
rot: rotation (tor)
rout: routine
RP:
 radial pulse
 refractory period
 respiratory rate: pulse rate
  (index)
 retrograde pyelography
R-5-P: ribose-5-phosphate
RPCF: Reiter protein complement
 fixation test (test for syphilis)
RPF:
 relaxed pelvic floor
 renal plasma flow
RPG: radiation protection guide
RPh: Registered Pharmacist
RPL-12: infectious lymphoid neo-
 plasm (of chickens)
rpm: revolutions per minute
RPMI: Roswell Park Memorial
 Institute
RPP: retropubic prostatectomy
RPPR: red cell precursor pro-
 duction rate
RPR: rapid plasma reagin (test)
RPS: renal pressor substance
rps: revolutions per second
RPT: Registered Physical
 Therapist
Rpt: report
RQ:
 recovery quotient
 respiratory quotient
R&R: rate and rhythm (of pulse)
RR:
 radiation reaction (cells)
 radiation response
 recovery room
 respiratory rate
 Riva-Rocci (sphygmomano-
  meter)
RRC:
 routine respiratory care
 Royal Red Cross
RR&E: round, regular and equal
 (with reference to pupils of
 eyes)
RRL: Registered Record Librarian
rRNA: ribosomal ribonucleic acid

RRP: relative refractory period
RRT: resazurin reduction time
RS:
 Rauwolfia serpentina
 reading of standard
 recipient's serum
 reinforcing stimulus
 resorcinol-sulphur
 respiratory syncytial (virus)
 response to stimulus (ratio)
 review of symptoms
 Reye's syndrome
 Ringer's solution
RSA:
 rabbit serum albumin
 right sacro-anterior (position of
  fetus)
RSB: Regimental Stretcher-
 Bearer
RScA: right scapuloanterior
rsch: research
RSCN: Registered Sick Children's
 Nurse
RScP: right scapuloposterior
 (position of fetus)
RSIVP: rapid sequence intraven-
 ous pyelogram
RSL: right sacrolateral (position of
 fetus)
RSM: Royal Society of Medicine
RSNA: Radiological Society of
 North America
RSO: Resident Surgical Officer
RSP: right sacroposterior
 (position of fetus)
RSPH: Royal Society for the
 Promotion of Health
RSPK: recurrent spontaneous
 psychokinesis
RSR: regular sinus rhythm
RSSE: Russian spring-summer
 encephalitis
RST:
 radiosensitivity testing
 right sacrotransverse (position
  of fetus)
RSTMH: Royal Society of Tropical
 Medicine and Hygiene
RSV:
 respiratory syncytial virus
 Rous sarcoma virus
RT:
 radiologic technologist

radiotherapy
radium therapy
reaction time
reading test
recreational therapy
reduction time
Registered Technician
  (American Registry of X-ray
  Technicians)
resistance transfer
respiratory therapy
room temperature
rt: right
RTA:
  renal tubule acidosis
  road traffic accident
Rtd: retarded
RTF:
  resistance transfer factor
  respiratory tract fluid
rtl: rectal
R test: reductase test
RTR:
  Recreational Therapist
    Registered
  red blood cell turnover rate
RU:
  rat unit
  reading of unknown
  right upper
  Roentgen unit
Ru: ruthenium (chemical symbol
  for)
rub: *ruber* (L) red
RUE: right upper extremity
RU-EF-Tb: isoniazid
RUI: Royal University of Ireland
RUL:
  right upper eyelid
  right upper lobe (of lung)
RUO: right ureteral orifice
RUOQ: right upper outer
  quadrant (site of injection)
Ru5-P: ribulose-5-phosphate
rupt: rupture(d)
RUQ: right upper quadrant
RV:
  residual volume
  retroversion
  right ventricle
  rubella vaccine
RVA: renal vascular resistance
RVD: relative vertebral density

RVH: right ventricular hypertrophy
RVLG: right ventrolateral gluteal
  (site of injection)
RVO:
  Regional Veterinary Officer
  relaxed vaginal outlet
RVS:
  relative value scale or schedule
  reported visual sensation
RW: radiological warfare
R-W: Rideal-Walker (phenol coefficient test)
Rx:
  prescription
  recipe (L) take
  treatment or therapy

S

S:
  sacral (in vertebral formulas)
  saline
  saturated(ion)
  section
  sedimentation coefficient
  sensation
  sensitive
  signa, signetur (L) write, let it be
    written, label
  silicate
  single (marital status)
  singular
  smooth (with reference to
    colonies of bacteria)
  soft (with reference to diet)
  soluble
  solute
  space
  special preparations necessary
    for test
  spherical
  spherical lens
  stimulus
  subject (of an experiment)
  substrate
  sulphur (chemical symbol for)
  supravergence
  surgeon(ery)
  Svedberg unit of sedimentation
    coefficient
  synthesis (of DNA in cell cycle)

s:
scruple (apothecaries)
second (unit of time)
section
see
semis (L) half
sensation
series
sign(ed)
singular
sinister (L) left
son

Σ:
sigma (eighteenth letter of
Greek alphabet)
sum
euphemistic abbreviation for
syphilis

s-: symmetric isomer

s: *sine* (L) without

S1, S2, etc: first sacral nerve,
second sacral nerve, etc.

S1: first heart sound

S2: second heart sound

S_x: symptoms or signs

SA:
sarcoma
secundum artem (L) according
to the art
serum albumin
soluble in alkaline solution
specific activity
surface area
sustained action (with reference
to drugs)

S-A:
sino-atrial (node)
sino-auricular

Sa: samarium (chemical symbol
for)

sa: *secundum artem* (L) according
to art, by skill

S&A: sugar and acetone

SAB: Society of American
Bacteriologists

sacc: cogwheel (respiration)

SACH: Small Animal Care
Hospital

SAD: sugar, acetone, diacetic acid
(test)

SAFA: soluble antigen fluorescent
antibody (test)

SAH: subarachnoid haemorrhage

SAICAR: amino-imidazole-N-
succinocarboxamine

Sal: *Salmonella*

sal:
salicylate
secundum artis legis (L) according to the rules of art

salicyl: salicylate

Salm: *Salmonella*

SAM: sex arousal mechanism

SAMA: Student American Medical
Association

SAMI: socially acceptable monitor-
ing instrument

SAN: sinoatrial node

Sanat: sanatorium

sanit:
sanitarium
sanitation(ary)

S-A node: sinotrial node

sapon: saponification

SAR:
sexual attitude reassessment
structure activity relationship
(dentistry)

Sar: sulpharsphenamine

SAS: sterile aqueous suspension

SAT:
satellite
School Ability Test (psychology)
sine acido thymonucleinico (L)
without thymonucleic acid

sat: saturated

sat'd: saturated

SATL: surgical Achilles tendon
lengthening

satn: saturation

sat sol: saturated solution

SAU: statistical analysis unit

SB:
Bachelor of Science
shortness of breath
Stanford-Binet (intelligence
test)
stillbirth

Sb:
stibium (chemical symbol for (L)
antimony
strabismus

SBA: sick bay attendant (Navy)

SBE:
shortness of breath on exertion
subacute bacterial endocarditis

SBG: selenite brilliant green
SBNS: Society of British Neurological Surgeons
SBOM: soy bean oil meal
SBP:
   steroid-binding plasma (protein)
   systolic blood pressure
SBR:
   strict bed rest
   styrene-butadiene rubber
SBStJ: Serving Brother, Order of
   St John of Jerusalem
SBTI: soy bean trypsin inhibitor
SC:
   closure of semilunar valves
   sacrococcygeal
   science(tific)
   scilicet (L) namely
   scrupulus (L) scruple
   self-care
   service connected
   sex chromatin
   sick call
   sickle cell
   silicone coated
   stimulus, conditioned
   subcutaneous
   sugar coated
S-C: sickle cell haemoglobin C
   disease
Sc:
   scandium (chemical symbol for)
   scapula
sc: without correction
SCA: sperm-coating antigen
Scand: Scandinavian
SCAT:
   School and College Ability test
   sheep-cell agglutination test
scat: *scatula* (L) box
scat orig: *scatula originalis* (L)
   original package: manufacturer's package and
   label
SCB: strictly confined to bed
SCC:
   Services for Crippled Children
   squamous cell carcinoma
ScD: Doctor of Science
ScDA: *scapuladextra anterior* (L)
   right scapulo-anterior
   (position of fetus)
ScDP: *scapuladextra posterior* (L)

   right scapuloposterior
   (position of fetus)
SCE: subacute bacterial endocar-
   ditis
SCG: sodium cromoglycate
SChE: serum cholinesterase
SCI:
   Science Citation Index
   Science of Creative Intelligence
   (Transcendental Meditation)
Sci: science(tific)
SCID: severe combined immune
   deficiency
SCIPP: sacrococcygeal to inferior
   pubic point
SCL: scleroderma
ScLA: *scapulolaeva anterior* (L)
   left scapulo-anterior (position
   of fetus)
Scler: sclerosis
ScLP: *scapulolaeva posterior* (L)
   left scapuloposterior (pos-
   ition of fetus)
SCM: State Certified Midwife
SCN: potassium thiocyanate
SCOP: scopolamine
scp: spherical candle power
scr: scruple
SCRAP: Simple Complex
   Reaction-Time Apparatus
SCS: Society of Clinical Surgery
SCT: sugar-coated tablet
SCU: Special Care Unit
SCUBA: self-contained under-
   water breathing apparatus
SCV: smooth, capsulated, virulent
   (with reference to bacteria)
SD:
   septal defect
   skin dose
   spontaneous delivery
   standard deviation
   steptodornase
   sudden death
   systolic discharge
S-D: sickle cell haemoglobin D
   (disease)
Sd: stimulus drive (psychology)
S^d: stimulus, discriminative
SDA:
   sacrodextra anterior (L) right
   sacro-anterior (position of
   fetus)

specific dynamic action (of foods)

succinic dehydrogenase activity

SDC: succinyldicholine

SDE: specific dynamic effect

SDF: slow death factor

SDH: sorbitol dehydrogenase

SDP: *sacrodextra posterior* (L) right sacroposterior (position of fetus)

SDS:
School Dental Service
sodium dodecyl sulphate
Specific Diagnosis Service

Sds: sounds

SDT: *sacrodextra transversa* (L) right sacrotransverse (position of fetus)

SE:
saline enema
sanitary engineering
sphenoethmoidal (suture)
spherical equivalent
stage of exhaustion (in GAS)
standard error

Se: selenium (chemical symbol for)

SEA: spontaneous electrical activity (physiology)

SEA: sheep erythrocyte agglutination (test)

SEBM: Society of Experimental Biology and Medicine

SEC: soft elastic capsules

sec:
second (unit of time)
secondary
secretary
section(s)

sect: section

SED: skin erythema dose

sed:
sedes (L) stool
sedimentation

sed rate: sedimentation rate

sed time: sedimentation time

SEG: sonoencephalogram

segm: segmented

segs: segmented neutrophils (polymorphonuclear leucocytes)

SEM:
scanning electron microscope

standard error of mean

sem:
semen (L) seed
semi, semis (L) one-half
seminal

semidr: *semidrachma* (L) half a drachm

semih: *semihora* (L) half an hour

sem ves: seminal vesicle

SEN: State Enrolled Nurse

sen: sensitive

SENS: sensitivities test

SEP: somatosensory evoked potential

separ: *separatum* (L) separately

sept: *septem* (L) seven

seq: *sequela* (L) that which follows

seq luce: *sequenti luce* (L) the following day

SER: service

sER: smooth endoplasmic reticulum

Ser: serine

ser: series, serial

ser sect: serial sections

serv:
serva (L) keep, preserve
services

SES: socioeconomic status

sesquih: *sesquihora* (L) an hour and a half

sex: sexual

s expr: *sine expressione* (L) without expressing or pressing

SF:
scarlet fever
seminal fluid
serum fibrinogen
sodium azide, fecal (medium)
spinal fluid
Streptococcus faecalis
stress formula
sulphation factor (of blood serum)
Sweberg flotation (unit)
synovial fluid

SFC: spinal fluid count

SFL: Sexual Freedom League

SFO: subfornical organ

SFW: shell fragment wound

SG:
Sachs-Georgi (test)

soluble gelatin (with reference to capsules)
Surgeon General
sg: specific gravity
s-g: *subgenus* (L) subgenus
s-gg: *subgenera* (L) subgenera
SGO: Surgeon General's Office
SGOT: serum glutamic oxalo-acetic transaminase
SGP: Society of General Physiologists
SGPT: serum glutamic pyruvic transaminase
S-Gt: Sachs-Georgi test
SGV: salivary gland virus
SH:
serum hepatitis
social history
somatotrophic (growth) hormone
sulphydryl
surgical history
Sh:
sheep (in veterinary medicine)
Shigella (bacteriology)
sh:
short
shoulder
S&H: speech and hearing
SHBD: serum X-hydroxy-butyrate dehydrogenase
SHBG: sex hormone-binding globulin
SHCO: sulphated hydrogenated castor oil
SHDI: supraoptical hypophysial diabetes insipidis
SHG diet: Sauerbruch, Herrmannsdorfer, Gerson diet (in TB)
SHHD: Scottish Home and Health Department
Shig: *Shigella*
SHMO: Senior Hospital Medical Officer
SHO: Senior House Officer
SHS: Sayer head sling
SI:
sacroiliac
saline injection (abortion)
saturation index
serum iron
soluble insulin

Système Internationale d'Unités (International System of Units)
Si: silicon (chemical symbol for)
SIA: synalbumin-insulin antagonism
sibs: siblings
sic:
siccus (L) dry
thus so; as stated
SICSVA: sequential impaction cascade sieve volumetric air (sampler)
SIDS: sudden infant death syndrome
SIECUS: Sex Information and Education Council of the United States
Sig: sigmoidoscopy
sig: *signa, signetur* (L) write, let it be written, label
sig n pro: *signa nomine proprio* (L) label with the proper name
SIM:
Society of Industrial Microbiology
sulphide, indole, motility (medium)
simp: *simplex* (L) simple
sine: sinusoidal
sing:
singular (one)
singulorum (L) of each
SINR: Swiss Institute of Nuclear Research
si n val: *si non valet* (L) if it does not answer *or* is not of value
si op sit: *si opus sit* (L) if necessary
SIRA: British Scientific Instrument Research Association
SIS: sterile injectable suspension
SISI: short increment sensitivity index
si vir perm: *si vires permitant* (L) if the strength will permit
SIW: self-inflicted wound
SJR: Shinawara-Jones-Reinhart (unit)
SK: streptokinase
SKAT: Sex Knowledge and Aptitude (test)
SKF: Smith, Kline, and French

SKI: Sloan-Kettering Institute
SL:
  satellite-like
  sensation level (of hearing)
  small lymphocytes
  sodium lactate
  solidified-liquid
  streptolysin
  sublingual

sl:
  secuandum legem (L) accord-
    ing to the rules
  sensu lato (L) in the broad sense
  slightly
SLA: *sacrolaeva anterior* (L) left
    sacroanterior (position of
    fetus)
SLB: short leg brace
SLD: serum lactate dehydro-
    genase
SLE:
  Saint Louis encephalitis
  systemic lupus erythematosus
SLP: *sacrolaeva posterior* (L) left
    sacroposterior (position of
    fetus)
SLR:
  straight leg raising
  Streptococcus lactis R
    (factor)
SLS: segment long-spacing (col-
    lagen fibres)
SLT: *sacrolaeva transversa* (L) left
    sacrotransverse (position of
    fetus)
SITr: silent treatment
SM:
  Master of Science
  Sexual Myths (scale)
  simple mastectomy
  somatomedin
  streptomycin
  sustained medication
  systolic murmur
Sm: samarium (chemical symbol
    for)
sm: small
SMA: sequential multiple analysis
SMAF: smooth muscle activating
    factor
sm an: small animal
Smb: standard mineral base
    (medium)

SMC:
  Scientific Manpower Com-
    mission
  succinylmonocholine
SMD: submanubrial dullness
SMDC: sodium-N-methyl
    dithiocarbamate dihydrate (a
    soil sterilizant)
SMI: Senior Medical Investigator
SMO:
  Medical Officer of Schools
  Senior Medical Officer (navy)
SMOH:
  Society of Medical Officers of
    Health
  Senior Medical Officer of Health
SMON: subacute myelo-
    opticoneuropathy
SMR:
  somnolent metabolic rate
  standard mortality rate
  submucuous resection
SMSA: Standard Metropolitan
    Statistical Areas
SMWDSep: single, married,
    widowed, divorced, separated
SN:
  serum neutralization
  Staff Nurse
  Student Nurse
  subnormal
S/N: signal to noise (ratio)
Sn: *stannum* (L) tin (chemical
    symbol for)
sn: *secundum naturam* (L) accord-
    ing to nature
SNDO: Standard Nomenclature of
    Diseases and Operations
SNF: Skilled Nursing Facility
SNM: Society of Nuclear Medicine
SNMT: Society of Nuclear Medical
    Technologists
SNOP: Standard Nomenclature of
    Pathology (College of Ameri-
    can Pathologists)
SNS:
  Society of Neurological
    Surgeons
  sympathetic nervous system
SO:
  salpingo-oophorectomy
  spheno-occipital (synchon-
    drosis)

standing orders
superior oblique (muscle)
supraoptic (nucleus)
so: south
SO₄: sulphate
S&O: salpingo-oophorectomy
SOAP: subjective, objective assessment and plan
SOB:
 see order blank
 shortness of breath
 suboccipitobregmatic
soc: social
SocSec: Social Security
sod: sodium
SOL: space-occupying lesion
sol:
 soluble
 solutio (L) a solution
solidif: solidification
soln: solution
solv:
 solve (L) dissolve
 solvent
somat: somatic
SOMOS: Society of Military Orthopaedic Surgeons
SOP: standard operating procedure
s op s: *si opus sit* (L) if necessary
S-O-R: stimulus-organism-response
Sorb D: sorbitol dehydrogenase
sos: *si opus sit* (L) if necessary
SOTT: synthetic medium old tuberculin trichloracetic acid precipitated
SP:
 sacrum to pubis
 stool preservative (Hajna)
 suprapubic
S/P: status post
Sp:
 spine (esp. spine of scapula)
 Spirillum
 summation potential
sp:
 space
 species (taxonomy)
 specific
 spinal
 spiritus (L) spirit
Span: Spanish

SPC: salicylamide, phenacetin (acetophenetidin) and caffeine
SPCA: serum prothrombin conversion accelerator (Factor VII), proconvertin
sp cd: spinal cord
spec:
 special
 specialist
 specific
 specimen
spec gr: specific gravity
specif: specification
SPF:
 specific pathogen free
 spectrophotofluorometer
sp fl: spinal fluid
sp gr: specific gravity
sph:
 spherical
 spherical lens
sp ht: specific heat
SPI: serum precipitable iodine
sp indet: *species indeterminata* (L) species indeterminate
sp inquir: *species inquirendae* (L) species of doubtful status
spir:
 spiral
 spiritual
 spiritus (L) spirit
spiss: *spissus* (L) dried
SPK: spinnbarkeit (with reference to cervical mucus)
SPL: sound pressure level
sp n: *species novum* (L) new species
sp nov: *species novum* (L) new species
spon: spontaneous
SPP:
 Sexuality Preference Profile
 suprapubic prostatectomy
spp: species (plural)
SPPS: stable plasma protein solution
SPR: Society for Psychical Research
SPS: sulphite polymixin sulphadiazine (agar)
spt: *spiritus* (L) spirit
SQ: subcutaneous

sq: square

sq cell ca: squamous cell carcinoma

sqq: *sequentia* (L) and following

SQ3R: survey, question, read, review, recite (psychology)

SR:
sarcoplasmic reticulum
secretion rate
sedimentation rate
senior
Senior Registrar
sensitization response
sex ratio
sigma reaction
sinus rhythm
soluble, repository (with reference to penicillin)
stage of resistance (in general adaptation syndrome)
stimulus-response
stomach rumble
systems review

Sr: strontium (chemical symbol for)

[85]Sr: radioactive strontium

SRA: Science Research Associates

SRaw: specific resistance, airway

SRBC: sheep red blood cells

SR cells: sensitization response cells (in vaginal smears)

SRD: soluble, repository, plus dihydrostreptomycin (with reference to penicillin)

SRF: somatotrophin-releasing factor

SRN: State Registered Nurse

sRNA: soluble ribonucleic acid

SRS:
slow reacting substance
Social and Rehabilitation Service (HEW)

SRS-A: slow reacting substance of anaphylaxis

SRT:
sedimentation rate test
speech reception threshold

SS:
saline soak
saliva sample
saturated solution
serum sickness
Shigella and *Salmonella* (agar)
single-stranded (DNA)
soap suds
sparingly soluble
standard score (psychology)
sterile solution
suction socket

ss: *sensu stricto* (L) in the strict sense

ss (ss̄): *semis* (L) one half

SSA:
skin-sentizing antibodies
Social Security Administration
Smith surface antigen

SSCQT: Selective Service College Qualifying Test

SSCr: stainless steel crown (dentistry)

SSD: source-skin distance

SSE: soapsuds enema

SSI: supplemental security income

SSP: supersensitivity perception

SSPE: subacute sclerosing panencephalitis

SSS:
specific soluble substance (polysaccharide hapten)
sterile saline soak

sss: *stratum super stratum* (L) layer upon layer

SSStJ: Serving Sister, Order of St John of Jerusalem

s str: *sensu stricto* (L) in the strict sense

SSU: self-service unit

ssv: *sub signo veneni* (L) under a poison label

ST:
esotropia (with l or r)
sedimentation time
skin test
slight trace
standardized test (psychology)
station
stimulus
surface tension
survival time

ST 37: hexylresorcinol

St: subtype

st:
stet, stent, (L) let it stand, let them stand

stabs: band cells (non-segmented polymorphonuclear leucocytes)

standard: standardization(ized)

StanPsych: Standard Psychiatric (nomenclature)

Staph: *Staphylococcus*

stat:
statim (L) at once, immediately
statistics

Stb: stillborn

STD:
sexually transmitted disease
skin test dose
standard test dose

std: standard(ized)

Stereo: stereogram

STH: somatotrophic (growth) hormone

STI: serum trypsin inhibitor

STIA: Scientific, Technological, and International Affairs

stillat: *stillatim* (L) by drops or in small quantities

stillb: stillborn

stimn: stimulation

STL: swelling, tenderness, limitation (of movement)

STP:
2, 5-dimethoxy-4-methyl-amphetamine (DOM)
standard (normal) temperature and pulse
standard temperature and pressure

STPD: standard temperature and pressure, dry

Strep: *Streptococcus*

struct: structural

STS:
serological test for syphilis
standard test for syphilis

STT: sensitization test

STU: skin test unit

SU:
sensation unit
strontium unit

su: *sumat* (L) let him take

SUA: serum uric acid

subac: subacute

subcrep: subcrepitant

subcut: subcutaneous(ly)

sub fin coct: *sub finem coctionis* (L) towards the end of boiling

subgen: *subgenus* (L) subgenus

subling: sublingual

submand: submandibular

subq: subcutaneous (injection)

subsp: *subspecies* (L) subspecies

substd: substandard

suc: *succus* (L) juice

Succ: succinate

suf: sufficient

sulph: sulphate

sulpha: sulphonamide

sum: *sume, sumantur* (L) take, let it be taken

sum tal: *sumat talem* (L) take one like this

sup:
superior
supination
supra (L) above, superior

supp: suppository

suppl: supplement(ary)

suppos: suppository

supra cit: *supra citato* (L) cited above

supt: superintendent

Surg:
surgeon
surgery(ical)

SUS: supressor sensitive

susp: suspension

SV:
sarcoma virus
satellite virus
scalp vein
simian virus
sinus venosus
snake venom
stroke volume

sv:
single vibrations
spiritus vini (L) alcoholic spirit

SVC: superior vena cava

SVCS: superior vena cava syndrome

SVI: stroke volume index

svr: *spiritus vini rectificatus* (L) rectified spirit of wine, alcohol

svt: *spiritus vini tenuis* (L) proof spirit

SW: Social Worker

Sw: swine (in veterinary medicine)
SWD: short wave diathermy
SWI: stroke work index
SWR: serum Wassermann reaction
SWS: slow wave sleep
Sx: symptoms or signs
sym:
  symmetry(ical)
  symptoms
symb: symbol(ic)
sympath: sympathetic
sympt: symptoms
syn: synonym
synd: syndrome
synth: synthetic
syph:
  syphilis
  syphilology(ist)
syr: *syrupus* (L) syrup
sys: system(ic)
syst:
  systemic
  systolic
syst m: systolic murmur
Sz: seizure

T

T:
  tau (Greek letter)
  temperature
  temporary
  tension (esp. intra-ocular)
  tera (prefix)
  thoracic
  thymine
  thymus-derived (lymphocyte)
  thyroid
  tidal gas (respiration)
  topical (with reference to administration of drugs)
  total
  toxicity
  transition point
  transmittance (symbol for, in spectrophotometry)
  transverse
  tumour
  type

t:
  temporal
  ter (L) three times
  terminal
  time
τ: tau (19th letter of the Greek alphabet)
  symbol for life (time) of radioactive isotope
$T\frac{1}{2}$: symbol for half-life (time) of radioactive isotope
T_1, T_2, etc: first thoracic vertebra, second thoracic vertebra, etc.
T_3: triiodothyronine
T_4: thyroxine
T+1, T+2, etc.: Symbols indicating stages of increased intraocular tension.
T−1, T−2, etc.: Symbols indicating stages of decreased intraocular tension
T-1824: Evans blue
TA:
  Teaching Assistant
  temperature, axillary
  toxin-antitoxin
  Transactional Analysis
  transaldolase
  tryptophane acid (reaction)
  tuberculin, alkaline
Ta: tantalum (chemical symbol for)
T&A:
  tonsillectomy and adenoidectomy
  tonsillitis and adenoiditis
  tonsils and adenoids
TAB: typhoid, paratyphoid A, and paratyphoid B (vaccine)
tab: *tabella* (L) a tablet
TABC: typhoid-paratyphoid A, B and C vaccine
TABT: combined TAB vaccine, tetanus toxoid
TABTD: combined TAB vaccine, tetanus toxoid and diphtheria toxoid
TACE: chlorotrianisene
TAF:
  toxoid-antitoxin floccules
  Tuberculin Albumose-frei (Ger) albumose-free tuberculin
  tumour angiogenesis factor

TAH: total abdominal hysterectomy

tal: *talis* (L) such a one

TAM:
thermoacidurans agar modified
toxoid-antitoxin mixture

TAM$_E$: tosyl-arginine methyl ester

TAMIS: Telemetric Automated Microbial Identification System

TAN: total ammonia nitrogen

tan: tangent

TANS: Territorial Army Nursing Service

TAO: triacetyloleandomycin

T'ASE: tryptophane synthetase

TAT:
Thematic Apperception Test
toxin-antitoxin

TB:
thymol blue (an indicator)
total base
tracheal bronchiolar (region)
tracheobronchitis
tubercle bacillus
tuberculosis

Tb: terbium (chemical symbol for)

TBA:
tertiary butyl acetate
thiobarbituric acid
tubercle bacillus
tuberculosis

TBE: tuberculin bacillen emulsion

TBG: thyroxine-binding globulin

TBGP: total blood granulocyte pool

TBI:
p-aminobenzaldehyde thiosemicarbazone
tooth brushing instruction (dentistry)
total body irradiation

TBLC: term birth, living child

TBM: tuberculous meningitis

TBP:
bithionol
testosterone-binding protein
thyroxine-binding protein
tributyl phosphate

TBPA: thyroxine-binding pre-albumin

tbs: tablespoon

tbsp: tablespoon

TB- Vis: isoniazid

TBW:
total body water
total body weight

TC:
tetracycline (antibiotic)
thermal conductivity
thoracic cage
thyrocalcitonin
tissue culture
to contain
total cholesterol
tuberculin, contagious
type and crossmatch

Tc:
technetium (chemical symbol for)

T&C: turn and cough

TCA:
tricalcium aluminate
tricarboxylic acid (cycle)
trichloroacetate
trichloroacetic acid

TCAP: trimethyl-cetyl-ammonium pentachlorphenate (a fungicide)

TCBS: thiosulphate citrate bile salts (agar)

TCC: thromboplastic cell component

TCD: tissue culture dose

TCE: tetrachloro-diphenyl-ethane (a mosquito larvicide)

TCESOM: trichlorethylene-extracted soybean-oil meal

TCH: turn, cough, hyperventilate

Tchg: teaching

Tchr: teacher

TCI: to come in (to hospital)

TCID: tissue culture infective dose

TCID$_{50}$: median tissue culture infective dose

TCP: tricreslyl phosphate (an antiesterase)

TCT:
calcitonin
thyrocalcitonin

TCu: copper T (an IUD)

TCV: thoracic cage volume

TD:
tetanus and diphtheria (toxoids)
thoracic duct
thymus dependent (cells)

timed disintegration
to deliver
torsion dystonia
total disability
treating distance
treatment or therapy
   discontinued
typhoid-dysentery
td: *ter die* (L) three times daily
TDD: Tuberculous Diseases
   Diploma
TDE: tetrachlorodiphenylethane
   (an insecticide) (SYN: *DDD*)
TDI: toluene diisocyanate
TDN : total digestible nutrients
TDS: temperature, depth, salinity
tds: *ter die sumendum* (L) to be
   taken three times a day
TDZ: thymus-dependent zone (of
   lymph node)
TE:
   tracheoesophageal
   trial (and) error
Te:
   tellurium (chemical symbol for)
   tetanus
T-e: SEE ET-3
TEA: tetraethylammonium
TEAB: tetraethylammonium
   bromide
TEAC: tetraethylammonium
   chloride
T&EC: Trauma and Emergency
   Center
tech: technical
TED: threshold erythema dose
TEE: tyrosine ethyl ester
TEM:
   transmission electron
     microscope
   triethylenemelamine
temp:
   temperature
   temporal
   temporary
temp dext: *tempus dextro* (L) to
   the right temple
temp sinist: *tempus sinistro* (L) to
   the left temple
TEN: total excretory (or excreted)
   nitrogen
TEPA: triethylenephosphoramide
TEPP: tetraethylpyrophosphate

ter:
   tere (L) rub
   tertiary
Terleu: tertiary leucine
term: terminal
ter sim: *tere simul* (L) rub together
TET: Teacher of Electrotherapy
tet: tetanus
TETRAC: tetraiodothyroacetic
   acid
TEV: talipes equinovarus
TF:
   tactile fremitus
   transfer factor
   tuberculin filtrate
   tuning fork
TFA: total fatty acids
TFN:
   total faecal nitrogen
TFNS: Territorial Force Nursing
   Service
TF/P: tubular fluid plasma
TFR: total fertility rate
TFS: testicular feminization
   hormone
TG:
   tetraglycine
   thyroglobulin
   triglyceride
Tg: type genus
TGE:
   transmissible gastroenteritis
   tryptone glucose extract (broth
     or agar)
TGT: thromboplastin generation
   test or time
TGY: tryptone (tryptophane peptone) glucose yeast (agar)
TH:
   tetrahydrocortisol
   thyroid hormone (thyroxine)
Th:
   thoracic
   thorax
   thorium (chemical symbol for)
THA: tetrahydroaminoacridine
THAM: trihydroxymethylamino-
   methane (tromethamine)
THC:
   tetrahydrocannabinol
   thiocarbanidin
THE: tetrahydrocortisone or
   tetrahydro E

theor: theoretical
ther:
  therapeutic
  therapy
  thermometer
ther ex: therapeutic exercise
THF:
  tetrahydrocortisone or
    tetrahydro F
  tetrahydrofolate
  tetrahydrofluorenone
  tetrahydrofuran
  thymic humoral factor
THFA:
  tetrahydrofurfuryl alcohol
  tetrahydrofolic acid
THM: total heme mass
Thor: thorax(ic)
THPA: tetrahydropteric acid
Thr: threonine
THRF: thyrotrophic hormone-
  releasing factor
Throm: thrombosis
THT: Teacher of Hydrotherapy
TI:
  thymus independent (cells)
  transverse diameter between
    ischia
  tricuspid insufficiency (incom-
    petence)
Ti: titanium (chemical symbol for)
TIA: transient ischaemia attack
TIBC: total iron-binding capacity
TIC: trypsin inhibitory capacity
tid: *ter in die* (L) three times daily
TIF: tumour inducing factor
TIG: tetanus immune globulin
tin: *ter in nocte* (L) three times
  nightly
tinc: tincture
tinct: tincture
TIP: translation inhibiting protein
TIRR: Texas Institute of Rehabili-
  tation and Research
TJ: triceps jerk
TK: transketolase
TKD: tokodynamometer
TKG: tokodynagraph
TL:
  terminal limen
  total lipids
  tubal ligation
Tl: thallium (chemical symbol for)

T-L: thymus-dependent
  lymphocyte
TLC:
  tender loving care
  thin-layer chromatography
  total lung capacity
TLD: thoracic lymph duct
TLE: thin-layer electrophoresis
TLS: testing the limits for sex (psychology)
TLV:
  threshold limit value
  total lung volume
TM:
  trade mark
  transport mechanism
  transport messenger
  tympanic membrane
T-M: Thayer-Martin (medium)
Tm:
  maximal tubular excretory
    capacity (of kidney)
  thulium (chemical symbol for)
TMA:
  tetramethylammonium
  trimethoxyphenyl amino-
    propane (a hallucinogen)
TM$_G$: maximum tubular reab-
  sorption rate (of kidney) for
  glucose
TME: Teacher of Medical Elec-
  tricity
TMJ: temporomandibular joint
TMMG: Teacher of Massage and
  Medical Gymnastics
Tm$_{PAH}$: maximum tubular excret-
  ory capacity (of kidney) for
  PAH
TMP:
  thymidine monophosphate
  transmembrane potentials
  trimethoprim
TMPD: tetramethyl-*p*-
  phenylinediamine
TMS: trimethylsilane
TMTD: tetramethylthiuram-
  disulphide
TMV: tobacco mosaic virus
TN: true negative
Tn: normal intraocular tension
Tng: training
TNM: tumour node (lymph) meta-
  stasis

TNT: trinitrotoluene
TNV: tobacco necrosis virus
TO:
original or old tuberculin (also
abbreviated OT)
target organ
telephone order
temperature, oral
tracheo-oesophageal
tuberculin ober (supernatant
portion
turnover (number)
to: *tinctura opii* (L) tincture of opium
TOCP: triorthocresylphosphate
TOE: tracheal-oesophageal
tol: tolerated
top: topically
TOPS: take off pounds sensibly
TOPV: trivalent oral poliovirus
vaccine
tox: toxic(ity)
TP:
temperature and pressure
terminal phalanx
testosterone proprionate
threshold potential
thymic polypeptide
toilet paper
total protein
transforming principle
(bacteriology)
Treponema pallidum
triphosphate
true positive
tuberculin precipitation
TPA: tannic acid, poly-
phosphomolybdic acid, amido
acid (staining technique)
TPB: tryptone phosphate broth
TPC:
thromboplastic plasma component
Treponema pallidum complement (fixation test)
TPCF: *Treponema pallidum* complement fixation (test)
TPD: thiamine propyl disulfide
TPEY: telluritepolymixin egg yolk
(agar)
TPF: thymus permeability factor
TPG: tryptophan peptone glucose
(broth)
TPI: *Treponema pallidum*

immobilization (test)
TPIA: *Treponema pallidum*
immune adherence (test)
TPN: triphosphopyridine
nucleotide
TPNH: triphosphopyridine
nucleotide, reduced form
TPO: tryptophan peroxidase
TPP: thiamine pyrophosphate
(diphosphothiamine)
TPR:
temperature, pulse, respiration
total peripheral resistance
TPT:
tetraphenyl tetrazolium (a histological stain)
total protein tuberculin
TR:
teaching and research
temperature, rectal
therapeutic radiology
tuberculin R (new tuberculin)
tuberculin residue
turbidity reducing
tr:
tincture
trace
traction
treatment
tremor
trach: trachea(otomy) (ostomy)
train: training
trans:
transaction
transfer
transverse
trans D: transverse diameter
transm: transmission
transpl: transplant(ation)
trans sect: transverse section
trau: trauma(tic)
TRBF: total renal blood flow
TRCH: tanned-red-cell
haemagglutination
treat: treatment
Trep: *Treponema*
TRF: thyrotrophin releasing factor
trg: training
TRH: thyrotrophin-releasing
hormone
TRI: total response index (psychology)
TRIAC: triiodothyroacetic acid

TRIC: trachoma inclusion conjunctivitis
trid: *triduum* (L) three days
TRIS: *tris* (hydroxymethyl) aminomethane
TRIT: triiodothyronine
trit: *tritura* (L) triturate
tRNA: transfer ribonucleic acid
troch: trochiscus, troche (a lozenge)
Trop Med: tropical medicine
TRP:
  total refractory period
  tubular reabsorption of phosphate
TrPl: treatment plan
TRSV: tobacco ringspot virus
TRT: treatment
TRU: turbidity reducing unit
Try: tryptophan
TS:
  temperature sensitive
  terminal (or greater) sensation
  test solution
  thoracic surgery
  total solids
  toxic substance
  transsexual
  tricuspid stenosis
  triple strength
  tubular (tracheal) sound
  tumour specific
T/S: thyroid: serum (radioiodide ratio)
TSA:
  tumour specific antigen
  toluene sulphonic acid (test)
TSD: target skin distance
T sect: transverse or cross section
T-set: tracheotomy set
TSH: thyroid-stimulating (thyrotophic) hormone
TSH-RF: thyroid-stimulating hormone-releasing factor
TSI: triple sugar (lactose, glucose, sucrose) iron (agar)
TSN: tryptophan peptone sulphide neomycin (agar)
TSP: total serum protein
tsp: teaspoon
TSR: testosterone sterilized (female) rat
TSSU: theatre sterile supply unit

TSTA: tumour specific transplantation antigen
TSU: triple sugar urea (agar)
TT:
  tablet triturate
  tetanus toxoid
  tetrathionate (Broth)
  thymol turbidity
  transit time (of blood through heart and lungs)
  tuberculin tested (milk)
TTC: triphenyltetrazolium chloride
TTH: thyrotrophic hormone (SEE *TSH*)
TTO: to take out
TTP: thrombotic thrombocytopenic purpura
TTPA: triethylene thiophosphoramide
TU:
  toxic unit
  transmission unit
  tuberculin unit
  turbidity unit
tuberc: tuberculosis
TUD: total urethral discharge
TUR: transurethral resection (of prostate)
turb: turbid(ity)
TURP: transurethral resection of the prostate
turp: turpentine
tus: *tussis* (L) cough
TV:
  tetrazolium violet
  tidal volume
  total volume
  transvestite
  Trichomonas vaginalis
  tuberculin volutin
TVC: triple voiding cystogram
TVD: transmissible virus dementia
TVF: tactile vocal fremitus
TVL: tenth value layer (with reference to radiation)
TVU: total volume urine (in twenty-four hours)
TW: total body water
TWA: time weighted average
TWE: tap water enema
TWSb: antimony dimercaptosuccinate

TX:
  treatment
  tuberculin (within cells of body)
Tx: treatment
Ty: type
Tymp:
  tympanicity (with reference to auscultation of chest)
  tympany(ic)
tymp memb: tympanic membrane
typ: typical
Tyr: tyrosine
Tz: tuberculin zymoplastiche (symbol for)
Tzn: total oestrogens after Zn-HCl treatment

U

U:
  unerupted (dentistry)
  unit
  unknown
  upper
  uracil
  uranium (chemical symbol for)
  uridine
  urology(ist)
^{235}**U:** radioactive uranium (chemical symbol for)
U/3: upper third (with reference to long bones)
UA:
  urinalysis
  uterine aspiration
ua: *usque ad* (L) up to, as far as
UAE: unilateral absence of excretion
UAN: uric acid nitrogen
UB: ultimobranchial (body)
UBA: undenatured bacterial antigen
UBI: ultra-violet blood irradiation
UC: urinary catheter
UCD: usual childhood diseases
UCG: urinary chorionic gonadotrophin
UCHD: usual childhood diseases
UCI: urinary catheter in
UCL: urea clearance (test)

UCO: urinary catheter out
UCR:
  unconditioned response
  usual, customary, and reasonable
UCS: unconditioned stimulus
Ucs: unconscious
UCV: uncontrolled variable
UD:
  ulnar deviation
  urethral discharge
  uridine diphosphate
ud: *ut dictum* (L) as directed
UDC:
  undeveloped countries
  usual diseases of childhood
UDPG: uridine diphosphate glucose
UDPGA: uridine diphosphate glucaronic acid
UDRP: uridine diribose phosphate
UE: upper extremity
u/ext: upper extremity
UFA: unesterified fatty acids
UG: urogenital
UGDP: University Group Diabetes Program
UGF: unidentified growth factor
UGI: upper gastrointestinal
UH: upper half
UHF: ultrahigh frequency
UHL: universal hypertrichosis lanuginosa
UIBC: unsaturated iron-binding capacity
UICC:
  Union International Contra le Cancrum (International Union against Cancer)
UIMC: International Union of Railway Medical Services
UK:
  United Kingdom
  unknown
UKAEA: United Kingdom Atomic Energy Authority
U&L: upper and lower
ULT: ultrahigh temperature (pasteurization)
ult: *ultimus* (L) ultimately, last
ult praes: *ultimum praescriptus* (L) last prescribed

UM:
 unmarried
 upper motor (neurons)
umb: umbilicus(ical)
UMNL: upper motor neuron lesion
UMP:
 uridine-5-monophosphate
 uridylic acid
UN:
 United Nations
 urea-nitrogen
uncomp: uncompensated
uncond: unconditioned
uncond ref: unconditioned reflex
UNCOR: uncorrected
UnCS: unconditioned stimulus
unct: *unctus* (L) smeared
undet ori: undetermined origin
UNESCO: United Nations
    Educational, Scientific, and
    Cultural Organization
ung: *unguentum* (L) ointment
UNICEF: United Nations Inter-
    national Children's
    Emergency Fund
unilat: unilateral
Univ: university
univ: universal
UNK: unknown
unof: unofficial
UNRRA: United Nations Relief
    and Rehabilitation Adminis-
    tration
UnS: unconditioned stimulus
uns:
 unsatisfactory
 unsymmetrical
unsat: unsaturated
unsym: unsymmetrical
UO: urinary output
UP: under proof
U/P: concentration in urine and
    plasma (e.g., glucose)
up ad lib: ambulatory (patient may
    walk)
UQ:
 ubiquinone
 upper quadrant
UR:
 unconditional response or
    reflex
 upper respiratory
 utilization review

Ur: urine
ur anal: urine analysis
ureth: urethra(al)
URF: uterine relaxing factor
urg: urgent
URI: upper respiratory infection
URO: uroporphyrin
uro-gen: urogenital
urol: urology(ist)
URQ: upper right quadrant
URT: upper respiratory tract
URTI: upper respiratory tract
    infection
US:
 ultrasound
 unconditioned stimulus
 United States
USA:
 United States of America
 United States Army
USAF: United States Air Force
USAH: United States Army
    Hospital
USAMEDS: United States Army
    Medical Service
USAN: United States Adopted
    Names (Council)
USASI: United States of America
    Standards Institute (formerly
    ASA, now ANST)
USBS: United States Bureau of
    Standards
USBuStand: United States
    Bureau of Standards
USCG: United States Coast Guard
USD: United States Dispensatory
USDHE&W: U.S. Department of
    Health, Education and Wel-
    fare
USHL: United States Hygenic
    Laboratory
USMC: United States Marine
    Corps
USMH: United States Marine
    Hospital
USN: United States Navy
USP: United States Pharma-
    copeia
USPHS: United States Public
    Health Service
USR: unheated serum reagin
    (test)
ust: *ustus* (L) burnt

USVB: United States Veterans Bureau

USVH: United States Veterans Hospital

UT: urinary tract

UTBG: unbound TBG

ut dict: *ut dictum* (L) as directed

utend: *utendus* (L) to be used

utend mor sol: *utendus more solito* (L) to be used in the usual manner

UTI: urinary tract infection

UTP: uridine triphosphate

UU: urine urobilinogen

UV: ultra-violet

U$_v$: Uppsula virus

UV/P: U = concentration of solute in urine; V = quantity of urine excreted in a unit of time; P = concentration of substance in plasma (ratio = clearance of the substance)

ux: wife

V

V:
coefficient of variation
Roman numeral five (5)
unipolar chest lead (in cardiography)
vaccinated
valve
vanadium (chemical symbol for)
variation
varnish (dentistry)
vein
velocity
ventilation
verbal
vertex
very
Vibrio (bacteriology)
violet (an indicator colour)
virulence
virus
vision
visual acuity
voice
volume

v:
vel (L) or
versus
very
vide (L) see
volt
von (Ger) of (used in names)

v-: vicinal isomer

VA:
vacuum aspiration
Veterans Administration
visual acuity

va: volt ampere

vac: vacuum

vacc: vaccination

VAD: Voluntary Aid Detachment

VAd: Veterans Administration

vag: vagina

VAH:
Veterans Administration Hospital
virilizing adrenal hyperplasia

VAKT: visual, association, kinaesthetic, tactile (with reference to reading)

Val: valine

var:
variation
variety

vasc: vascular

vas vit: *vas vitreum* (L) a glass vessel

VAT: ventricular activation time

VBOS: veronal buffered oxalated saline

VBS: veronal-buffered saline (medium)

VC:
colour vision
Veterinary Corps
vital capacity

VCC: vasoconstrictor centre

VCG: vectorcardiogram

VCI: volatile corrosion inhibitor

V-cillin: penicillin V

VCN: vancomycin hydrochloride, colistimethate sodium, nystatin (medium)

VCP: Veterinary Creolin-Pearson

VCR: vincristine

VCS: vasoconstrictor substance

VCU: voiding cystourethrogram

VD:
vapour density
venereal disease
virus diarrhoea
Vd: volume dead air space
vd: double vibrations (cycles)
VDA: visual discriminatory acuity
VDC: vasodilator centre
VDEL: Venereal Disease Experimental Laboratory
VDEM: vasodepressor material
VDG: venereal disease – gonorrhoea
VDH: valvular disease of heart
VDM: vasodepressor material
VDRL: Venereal Disease Research Laboratory
VDRT: Venereal Disease Reference Test (of Harris)
VDS:
vasodilator substance
venereal disease – syphilis
VE:
vaginal examination
ventilation
vesicular exanthema
visual efficiency
volume ejection
VEE: Venezuelan equine encephalomyelitis
vehic: *vehiculum* (L) vehicle
vel: velocity
veloc: velocity
VEM: vasoexcitor material
vent:
ventilator
ventricular
vent fib: ventricular fibrillation
ventr: ventral
ventric: ventricle (icular)
VEP: visual evoked potential
VER: visual evoked response
vert:
vertebra (al)
vertical
ves:
vesica (L) bladder
vesicular (with reference to chest sounds)
vesic: *vesicula* (L) a blister
vesp: *vesper* (L) evening
ves ur: *vesica urinaria* (L) urinary bladder

VET: vestigial testis (rat)
Vet:
veteran
veterinary
v et: *vide etiam* (L) see also
VetAdmin: Veterans Administration
VetSci: veterinary science
VF:
ventricular fibrillation
visual field
vocal fremitus
V factor: verbal comprehension factor (psychology)
VFDF: very fast death factor
Vfib: ventricular fibrillation
VG:
ventricular gallop
very good
VGH: very good health
VH:
Veterans Hospital
viral hepatitis
VI:
vaginal irrigation
variable interval (reinforcement)
virgo intacta
virulence
volume index
Vi: virginium (chemical symbol for)
VIA: virus inactivating agent
VIB: vocational interest blank
vib: vibration
VIBS: vocabulatory, information, block design, similarities (psychology)
VIC: vasoinhibitory centre
vic: *vices* (L) times
vid: *vide* (L) see
VIG: vaccinia immune globulin
vin: *vinum* (L) wine
VIP:
vasoactive intestinal polypeptide
vasoinhibitory peptide
very impor nt person
vir:
viridis (L) green
virulent
vis:
vision
visiting(or)

visc:
visceral
viscous(sity)
Vit: vitamin (when followed by a letter)
vit: vital
VitB₁: thiamine
VitB₂: riboflavin
VitB₃: nicotinamide
VitB₆: pyridoxine
VitB₁₂: cobalamine, cyanocobalamine
VitB₁₂ₕ: hydroxycobalamine
VitC: ascorbic acid
VitD₂: ergocalciferol
VitD₃: cholecalciferol (natural vitamin D)
VitE: tocopherol(s)
vitel: *vitellus* (L) yolk
VitG: riboflavin
VitH: biotin
VitK: coagulation vitamin, anti-haemorrhagic factor
vit ov sol: *vitello ovi solutus* (L) dissolved in yolk of egg
VitPP: nicotinamide; nicotinic acid
VitU: cabagin or anti-ulcer vitamin
vitr: *vitreum* (L) glass
viz: *videlicet* (L) namely
VJ: Vogel: Johnson (agar)
VL: vision, left
VLB: vincaleucoblastine (vinblastine)
VLDL: very low-density lipoprotein
VM:
vasomoter
vestibular membrane
viomycin
voltmeter
VMA: vanilmandelic acid
VMC: vasomotor centre
VMH: ventromedial hypothalamic (neurons)(nuclei)
VN:
virus neutralization
Visiting Nurse
Vocational Nurse
VNA: Visiting Nurse Association
VO: verbal order
voc: vocational
vocab: vocabulary
VOD:
venous occlusive disease

vision, right eye
vol:
volar
volatilis (L) volatile
volume(tric)
voluntary(eer)
vol/%: volume/per cent
volt: volatile(izes)
VOM: vinyl chloride monomer
VON: Victorian Order of Nurses (Canada)
VOS: vision left eye
vos: *vitello ovi solutus* (L) dissolved in yolk of egg
VP:
vapour pressure
venous pressure
Voges-Proskauer (test)
VPC:
ventricular premature beats
volume packed cells
VPP: viral porcine pneumonia
vps: vibrations per second
VR:
variable ratio (reinforcement)
venous return
ventilation rate
vision, right
vocal resonance
vocational rehabilitation
vr: ventral root (of a spinal nerve)
VRA: Vocational Rehabilitation Administration
VRI: virus respiratory infection
VRL: Virus Reference Laboratory
VRP: very reliable product
VS:
vaccination scar
verbal scale
vesicular sound (in auscultation of chest)
vesicular stomatitis
Veterinary Surgeon
vital sign
volumetric solution
Vs: *venaesectio* (L) venesection
vs:
single vibration(cycles)
versus
vibration seconds
vide supra (L) see above
VsB: *venaesectio brachii* (L) bleeding in the arm

VSD: ventricular septal defect
vsn: vision
VSS: vital signs stable
VT:
  tetrazolium violet (a histological stain)
  vacuum tuberculin
  vasotonin
Vt: tidal volume
V&T: volume and tension (of pulse)
VTE: vicarious trial and error (psychology)
V-test: Voluter test
VTG: volume thoracic gas
VTI: volume thickness index
VTOL: vertical take-off and landing
VU: very urgent
VV: vulva and vagina
vv:
  veins
  vice versa
v/v: percent volume (of solute) in volume (of solvent)
VW: vessel wall
Vx: vertex
V-Z: varicella-zoster

W

W:
  tungsten (*wolframium*) (chemical symbol for)
  water
  wehnelt (a unit of roentgen ray hardness)
  weight
  west
  white
  whole (response)
  widow(er)
  width
  word fluency (psychology)
w:
  watt
  week
  wife
  with

[185]W: radioactive tungsten
WA: when awake
WAC: Women's Army Corps
WAIS: Wechsler's Adult Intelligence Scale
WARF: Warfarin (a rodenticide)
Wass: Wassermann test
WB:
  washable base
  water bottle
  Wechsler-Bellevue scale
  weight-bearing
  wet-bulb
  whole blood
Wb: weber
WBC:
  white blood cell count
  white blood cells
WBE: whole body extract
WBR: whole body radiation
WBS: whole body scan
WBT: wet bulb temperature
WC:
  ward clerk
  water closet
  wheel chair
  white cell
  whooping cough
WD:
  Wallerian degeneration
  wet dressing
  wrist disarticulation
Wd: ward
w/d: well developed
wds: wounds
WDWN: well developed-well nourished
WEE: Western equine encephalitis
WEF: war emergency formula
W/F: white female
WFOT: World Federation of Occupational Therapists
wh:
  whispered
  white
WHAP: Woman's Health and Abortion Project
WHML: Wellcome Historical Medical Library
WHO: World Health Organization
whp: whirlpool
whr: watt hour

WHRC: World Health Research Centre

wid: widow(er)

WISC: Wechsler Intelligence Scale for Children

wk: week

WK dis: Wilson-Kimmelstiel disease

WL:
waiting list
Wallenstein Laboratory (medium)
wavelength

WL test: waterload test

WM: Ward Manager

W/M: white male

wm: whole mount (in microtechnic)

WMA: World Medical Association

WMR: World Medical Relief

WMSC: Women's Medical Specialists Corps

WMX: whirlpool, massage, exercise

w/n: well nourished

WNL: within normal limits

WO:
wash out
written order

W/O: water in oil (with reference to emulsions)

w/o: without

WP:
wet pack
whirlpool
working point

WPB: whirlpool bath

WPk:
Ward's mechanical tissue pack (dentistry)
wet pack

WPW: Wolff-Parkinson-White (syndrome)

WR:
Wassermann reaction
wrist

WRAT: Wide Range Achievement Test

WRC:
washed red cells
water-retention coefficient

W-response: whole response

WS: water soluble

wt: weight

W/V: weight of solute in volume of solvent

w/w: weight of solute in weight of solvent

WxB: wax bite

WxP: wax pattern

WZa: wide zone alpha (haemolysis)

X

X:
cross or transverse (with reference to selections)
extra
Kienboch's unit (of roentgen ray dosage)
magnification sign
Roman numeral ten (10)
sign of multiplication
times (multiplication sign)
unknown quantity (symbol for)
Xenopsylla (parasitology)

x: axis (of a cylindrical lens)

XA: xanthurenic acid

Xa: chiasma

X-A mixture: xylene-alcohol mixture (for killing insect larvae)

Xanth: xanthomatosis

X-chromosome: sex chromosome

Xe: xenon (chemical symbol for)

XES: X-ray energy spectrometer

X-factor: heme

XKO: not knocked out

XLD: xylose, lysine, desoxycholate (agar)

X-matching: cross matching

Xn: Christian

X-organ: neurosecretory organ in crustaceans

X-rays: roentgen rays

XT: exotropia (with L or R)

Xta: chiasmata

XU: excretory urogram

XX: normal female chromosome type

XY: normal male chromosome type

Xyl: xylose

Y

Y:
  yellow
  Yersinia
  young
  yttrium (chemical symbol for)
YADH: yeast alcohol dehydrogenase
YAG: yttrium aluminum garnet
Yb: ytterbium (chemical symbol for)
YCB: yeast carbon base
yd: yard
YE: yellow enzyme
YEH$_2$: reduced yellow enzyme
yel: yellow
YNB: yeast nitrogen base
y/o: years old
Y-organ: moulting gland in crustacea
YP: yield pressure
yr: year
yrs: years
ys: yellow spot (on retina)
yt: yttrium

Z

Z:
  atomic number (symbol for)
  impedence
  standard score (statistic)
  zero
  zone
  Zuckung (Ger) contraction
Z-disk: intermediate (Ger) *Zwischenscheibe* disk
ZE: Zollinger-Ellison (syndrome)
ZIG: zoster immunoglobulin
zI^a: Symbol for isotope with atomic number Z and atomic weight A
Zn: zinc (chemical symbol for)
Zool: zoology(ical)
ZPG: Zero Population Growth
ZPO: zinc peroxide
Zr: zirconium (chemical symbol for)
^{95}Zr: radioactive zirconium
Zz: *zingiber* (L) ginger
Z, Z^1, Z^{11}: increasing degrees of contraction

SYMBOLS

℥ : ounce
f℥ : fluid ounce
O : pint
lb : pound
℞ : recipe; take
M : misce, mix
āā āa : of each
A, Å : Angstrom unit
C′ : complement
c, c̄ : [*L. cum*] with
E₀ : electroaffinity
F₁ : first filial generation
F₂ : second filial generation
mμ : millimicron
μ**g** : microgram
mμg : millimicrogram
mEq : milliequivalent
mg : milligram
mg% : milligrams per cent
Qo₂ : oxygen consumption
m- : meta-
o- : ortho-
p- : para-
s̄s̄,ss : [*L. semis*]one-half
′ : foot; minute; primary accent, univalent
″ : inch; second; secondary accent; bivalent
′‴ : line (1/12 inch); trivalent
μ : micron
μμ : micromicron, pico
μμg : micromicrogram, picogram
+ : plus; excess; acid reaction; positive
− : minus; deficiency; alkaline reaction; negative
± : plus or minus; either positive or negative; indefinite

: number; following a number, pounds; fracture
÷ : divided by
× : multiplied by; magnification
= : equals
> : greater than; from which is derived
< : less than; derived from
√ : root; square root; radical
²√ : square root
³√ : cube root
∞ : infinity
: : ratio; "is to"
:: : equality between ratios; "as"
* : birth
† : death
° : degree
% : per cent
γ : microgram
λ : wavelength
σ : 1/1000 of a second; standard deviation
Σ : sum of
π : 3·1416 − ratio of circumference of a circle to its diameter
☐, ♂ : male
o, ♀ : female
⇌ : denotes a reversible reaction
↑ or ↗ : increase, increases
↓ or ↘ : decrease, decreases
→ : yields or causes
→ or ← : in a chemical equation, indicates direction of reaction

* Adapted from *Taber's Cyclopedic Medical Dictionary*, Twelfth Edition.
Symbols used in recording results of qualitative tests:
− : negative
± : very slight trace or reaction
+ : slight trace or reaction
+ + : trace or noticeable reaction
+ + + : moderate amount of reaction
+ + + + : large amount or pronounced reaction

ABBREVIATIONS OF TITLES OF THE PRINCIPAL MEDICAL JOURNALS

Titles consisting of only one word (e.g. *Lancet*) are not abbreviated and are therefore omitted from this list. Where confusion might arise between two journals with the same name, the place of publication is added in the abbreviation (e.g. *Nature, Lond.* and *Nature, Paris*). Nouns are spelt with a capital, adjectives with a small, initial letter. A full point is used after abbreviations but not after contractions.

The most commonly used methods of abbreviation of titles are the code introduced by the *World List of Scientific Periodicals* and the modified form of this code adopted by the International Standards Organization. The principal difference is that the first inserts a comma before place-names introduced to distinguish between otherwise identical titles, while the latter encloses such place-names within brackets, e.g. *Nature, Lond.* and *Nature (Lond.)*. The latter form is used in the list which follows as it is the style employed by the *Index Medicus* and *World Medical Periodicals*.

Acta allerg. (Kbh.)	*Acta allergologica.* København
Acta chir. scand.	*Acta chirurgica Scandinavica*
Acta endocr. (Kbh.)	*Acta endocrinologica.* København
Acta haemat. (Basel)	*Acta haematologica.* Basel
Acta med. scand.	*Acta medica Scandinavica*
Acta neurol. scand.	*Acta neurologica Scandinavica*
Acta obstet. gynec. scand.	*Acta obstetricia et gynaecologica Scandinavica*
Acta paediat. (Uppsala)	*Acta paediatrica.* Uppsala
Acta paediat. scand.	*Acta paediatrica Scandinavica*
Acta path. microbiol. scand.	*Acta pathologica et microbiologica Scandinavica*
Acta physiol. Scand.	*Acta physiologica Scandinavica*
Acta psychiat. Scand.	*Acta psychiatrica et neurologica Scandinavica*
Acta radiol. (Stockh.)	*Acta radiologica.* Stockholm
Albrecht v. Graefes Arch. Opthal.	*Albrecht v. Graefes Archiv für Ophthalmologie*
Amer. Heart J.	*American Heart Journal*
Amer. J. clin. Path.	*American Journal of Clinical Pathology*
Amer. J. dig. Dis.	*American Journal of Digestive Diseases*
Amer. J. Dis. Child.	*American Journal of Diseases of Children*
Amer. J. Epidem.	*American Journal of Epidemiology*
Amer. J. Gastroent.	*American Journal of Gastroenterology*
Amer. J. Hyg.	*American Journal of Hygiene*
Amer. J. Med.	*American Journal of Medicine*
Amer. J. med. Sci.	*American Journal of the Medical Sciences*
Amer. J. Obstet. Gynec.	*American Journal of Obstetrics and Gynecology*
Amer. J. Ophthal.	*American Journal of Ophthalmology*
Amer. J. Path.	*American Journal of Pathology*

Amer. J. Physiol.	American Journal of Physiology
Amer. J. Psychiat.	American Journal of Psychiatry
Amer. J. publ. Hlth	American Journal of Public Health
Amer. J. Roentgenol.	American Journal of Roentgenology
Amer. J. Surg.	American Journal of Surgery
Amer. J. trop. Med. Hyg.	American Journal of Tropical Medicine and Hygiene
Amer. J. vet. Res.	American Journal of Veterinary Research
Amer. Surg.	American Surgeon
Anim. Behav.	Animal Behaviour
Ann. Inst. Pasteur	Annales de l'Institut Pasteur
Ann. intern. Med.	Annals of Internal Medicine
Ann. N.Y. Acad. Sci.	Annals of the New York Academy of Sciences
Ann. Surg.	Annals of Surgery
Ann. thorac. Surg.	Annals of Thoracic Surgery
Antibiot. and Chemother.	Antibiotics and Chemotherapy
Arch. Biochem. Biophys.	Archives of Biochemistry and Biophysics
Arch. Derm. (Chicago)	Archives of Dermatology. Chicago
Arch. Dis. Childh.	Archives of Diseases in Childhood
Arch. gen. Psychiat.	Archives of General Psychiatry
Arch. ges. Virusforsch.	Archiv für die Gesamte Virusforschung
Arch. Gynäk.	Archiv für Gynäkologie
Arch. industr. Hlth	Archives of Industrial Health
Arch. intern. Med.	Archives of Internal Medicine
Arch. klin. Chir.	Archiv für klinische Chirurgie
Arch. Path.	Archives of Pathology
Arch. Pediat.	Archives of Pediatrics
Arch. Psychiat. Nervenkr.	Archiv für Psychiatrie und Nervenkrankheiten
Arch. Surg.	Archives of Surgery
Arth. and Rheum.	Arthritis and Rheumatism
Aust. dent. J.	Australian Dental Journal
Aust. J. Derm.	Australasian Journal of Dermatology
Aust. J. exp. Biol. med. Sci.	Australian Journal of Experimental Biology and Medical Science
Aust. paediat. J.	Australian Paediatric Journal
Aust. Radiol.	Australasian Radiology
Bact. Rev.	Bacteriological Reviews
Biochem. J.	Biochemical Journal
Biochem. Z.	Biochemische Zeitschrift
Biochim. biophys. Acta	Biochimica et biophysica Acta
Brit. dent. J.	British Dental Journal
Brit. Heart J.	British Heart Journal
Brit. J. Cancer	British Journal of Cancer
Brit. J. exp. Path.	British Journal of Experimental Pathology
Brit. J. Haemat.	British Journal of Haematology
Brit. J. Hosp. Med.	British Journal of Hospital Medicine
Brit. J. industr. Med.	British Journal of Industrial Medicine
Brit. J. Nutr.	British Journal of Nutrition
Brit. J. Ophthal.	British Journal of Ophthalmology
Brit. J. Pharmacol.	British Journal of Pharmacology
Brit. J. Psychiat.	British Journal of Psychiatry

Brit. J. Radiol.	British Journal of Radiology
Brit. J. Surg.	British Journal of Surgery
Brit. med. Bull.	British Medical Bulletin
Brit. med. J.	British Medical Journal
Bull. Hist. Med.	Bulletin of the History of Medicine
Bull. Hyg.	Bulletin of Hygiene
Bull. Johns Hopk. Hosp.	Bulletin of the Johns Hopkins Hospital
Bull. N.Y. Acad. Med.	Bulletin of the New York Academy of Medicine
Bull. Soc. méd. Paris	Bulletins et mémoires de la Société de Medicine de Paris
Bull. Wld Hlth Org.	Bulletin of the World Health Organization
Canad. J. Biochem.	Canadian Journal of Biochemistry and Physiology
Canad. med. Ass. J.	Canadian Medical Association Journal
Cancer Res.	Cancer Research
Cardiovasc. Res.	Cardiovascular Research
Cell Tiss. Kinet.	Cell and Tissue Kinetics
Chem. Abstr.	Chemical Abstracts
Clin. chim. Acta	Clinical chimica Acta
Clin. exp. Immunol.	Clinical and Experimental Immunology
Clin. Sci.	Clinical Science
C.R. Acad. Sci. (Paris)	Comptes rendus hebdomadaires des Séances de l'Académie des Sciences
C.R. Soc. Biol. (Paris)	Comptes rendus des Séances de la Société de Biologie
Dent. Practit. dent. Rec.	Dental Practitoner and Dental Record
Develop. Biol.	Developmental Biology
Dtsch. Arch. klin. Med.	Deutsches Archiv für klinische Medizin
Dtsch. med. Wschr.	Deutsche medizinische Wochenschrift
Electroenceph. clin. Neuro-physiol.	Electroencephalography and Clinical Neurophysiology
Epidem Mikrobiol.	Epidemiologija mikrobiologija, i infekciozni bolesti
Excerpta med. (Amst.)	Excerpta medica
Exp. Cell Res.	Experimental Cell Research
Exp. Med. Surg.	Experimental Medicine and Surgery
Exp. Molec. Path.	Experimental and Molecular Pathology
Fed. Proc.	Federation Proceedings
Guy's Hosp. Rep.	Guy's Hospital Reports
Hoppe-Seyl. Z. physiol. Chem.	Hoppe-Seylers Zeitschrift für physiologische Chemie
Hosp. Pract.	Hospital Practice
Indian J. med. Res.	Indian Journal of Medical Research
Indian med. Gaz.	Indian Medical Gazette
Int. J. Cancer	International Journal of Cancer
Invest. Radiol.	Investigative Radiology
Invest. Urol.	Investigative Urology
Irish J. med. Sci.	Irish Journal of Medical Science
Israel J. med. Sci.	Israel Journal of Medical Sciences
Jap. J. Med.	Japanese Journal of Medicine
Johns Hopk. med. J.	Johns Hopkins Medical Journal

J. Allergy	Journal of Allergy
J. Amer. chem. Soc.	Journal of the American Chemical Society
J. Amer. dent. Ass.	Journal of the American Dental Association
J. Amer. med. Ass.	Journal of the American Medical Association
J. Anat. (Lond.)	Journal of Anatomy. London
J. appl. Physiol.	Journal of Applied Physiology
J. Bact.	Journal of Bacteriology
J. biol. Chem.	Journal of Biological Chemistry
J. Bone Jt Surg.	Journal of Bone and Joint Surgery
J. Cell Biol.	Journal of Cell Biology
J. cell. comp. Physiol.	Journal of Cellular and Comparative Physiology
J. chem. Soc.	Journal of the Chemical Society
J. clin. Endocr.	Journal of Clinical Endocrinology
J. clin. Invest.	Journal of Clinical Investigation
J. clin. Path.	Journal of Clinical Pathology
J. dent. Res.	Journal of Dental Research
J. Endocr.	Journal of Endocrinology
J. exp. Med.	Journal of Experimental Medicine
J. gen. Microbiol	Journal of General Microbiology
J. gen. Physiol.	Journal of General Physiology
J. Hist. Med. allied Sci.	Journal of the History of Medicine and Allied Sciences
J. Hyg. (Camb.)	Journal of Hygiene. Cambridge
J. Immunol.	Journal of Immunology
J. Indian med. Ass.	Journal of the Indian Medical Association
J. infect. Dis.	Journal of Infectious Diseases
J. invest. Derm.	Journal of Investigative Dermatology
J. Lab. clin. Med.	Journal of Laboratory and Clinical Medicine
J. Laryng.	Journal of Laryngology and Otology
J. med. Sci	Journal of Medical Sciences
J. ment. Sci.	Journal of Mental Science
J. nat. Cancer Inst.	Journal of the National Cancer Institute
J. nerv. ment. Dis.	Journal of Nervous and Mental Disease
J. Neurophysiol.	Journal of Neurophysiology
J. Neurosurg.	Journal of Neurosurgery
J. Nutr.	Journal of Nutrition
J. Obstet. Gynaec. Brit. Cmwlth	Journal of Obstetrics and Gynaecology of the British Commonwealth
J. Parasit.	Journal of Parasitology
J. Path. Bact.	Journal of Pathology and Bacteriology
J. Pharmacol.	Journal of Pharmacology
J. Physiol. (Lond.)	Journal of Physiology. London
J. roy. micr. Soc.	Journal of the Royal Microscopical Society
J. thorac. cardiovasc. Surg.	Journal of Thoracic and Cardiovascular Surgery
J. thorac. Surg.	Journal of Thoracic Surgery
J. trop. Med. Hyg.	Journal of Tropical Medicine and Hygiene
Klin. Wschr.	Klinische Wochenschrift
Life Sci.	Life Sciences
Mayo Clin. Proc.	Mayo Clinic Proceedings

Med. Clin. N. Amer.	Medical Clinics of North America
Med. J. Aust.	Medical Journal of Australia
Med. Press	Medical Press
Med. Welt	Medizinische Welt
Meth. Cancer Res.	Methods of Cancer Research
Milit. Med.	Military Medicine
Münch. med. Wschr.	Münchener medizinische Wochenschrift
Nature (Lond.)	Nature. London
New Engl. J. Med.	New England Journal of Medicine
Nutr. Abstr. Rev.	Nutrition Abstracts and Reviews
Obstet. Gynec. Surv.	Obstetrical and Gynecological Survey
Obstet. and Gynec.	Obstetrics and Gynecology
Pflügers Arch. ges. Physiol.	Pflügers Archiv für die gesamte Physiologie
Pharm. J.	Pharmaceutical Journal
Pharmacol. Rev.	Pharmacological Reviews
Phil. Trans. B	Philosophical Transactions of the Royal Society, Series B
Physiol. Rev.	Physiological Reviews
Postgrad. Med.	Postgraduate Medicine
Postgrad. med. J.	Postgraduate Medical Journal
Presse méd.	Presse medicale
Proc. Mayo Clin.	Proceedings of the Staff Meetings of the Mayo Clinic
Proc. roy. Soc. B	Proceedings of the Royal Society, Series B
Proc. roy. Soc. Med.	Proceedings of the Royal Society of Medicine
Proc. Soc. exp. Biol. (N.Y.)	Proceedings of the Society for Experimental Biology and Medicine
Publ. Hlth Rep. (Wash.)	Public Health Reports. Washington
Quart. J. exp. Physiol.	Quarterly Journal of Experimental Physiology
Quart. J. Med.	Quarterly Journal of Medicine
Scand. J. Urol. Nephrol.	Scandinavian Journal of Urology and Nephrology
Schweiz. med. Wschr.	Schweizerische Medizinische Wochenschrift
Sci. Basis Med.	Scientific Basis of Medicine
Sem. Hôp. Paris	Semaine des hôpitaux de Paris
Ser. Haematol.	Series Haematologica
S. Afr. J. Surg.	South African Journal of Surgery
S. Afr. med. J.	South African Medical Journal
Surg. Gynec. Obstet.	Surgery, Gynaecology and Obstetrics
Surg. Clin. N. Amer.	Surgical Clinics of North America
Trans. roy. Soc. trop. Med. Hyg.	Transactions of the Royal Society of Tropical Medicine and Hygiene
Trop. Dis. Bull.	Tropical Diseases Bulletin
U.S. armed Forces med. J.	U.S. Armed Forces Medical Journal
Vet. Med.	Veterinary Medicine
Vet. Rec.	Veterinary Record
Virchows Arch. path. Anat.	Virchows Archiv für pathologische Anatomie

Wien. klin. Wschr.	*Wiener klinische Wochenschrift*
Wien. med. Wschr.	*Wiener medizinische Wochenschrift*
Wld Hlth Org. techn. Rep. Ser.	*World Health Organization Technical Report Series*
Wld Med.	*World Medicine*
Yale J. Biol. Med.	*Yale Journal of Biology and Medicine*
Z. Chem.	*Zeitschrift für Chemie*
Z. ges. exp. Med.	*Zeitschrift für die gesamte experimentelle Medizin*
Z. Hyg. Infekt.-Kr.	*Zeitschrift für Hygiene und Infektionskrankheiten*
Z. Immun.-Allergie-Forsch.	*Zeitschrift für Immunitäts-und Allergieforschung*
Z. klin. Chem.	*Zeitschrift für klinische Chemie und klinische Biochemie*
Z. klin. Med.	*Zeitschrift für klinische Medizin*
Zbl. Bakt.	*Zentralblatt für Bakteriologie*

SOME USEFUL SOURCE BOOKS

Abbrevs (A Dictionary of Abbreviations) (Stephenson), New York: Macmillan Co.

Acronyms, Initialisms and Abbreviations Dictionary (Crowley), 5th ed. Detroit, Mich.: Gale Research.

Allen's Dictionary of Abbreviations and Symbols. New York: Coward McCann.

American Druggist Blue Book, The. (Contains an extensive list of Latin abbreviations and their English equivalents.)

American Standard Abbreviations for Scientific and Engineering Terms. American Society of Mechanical Engineers.

Chamber's Technical Dictionary. London: Chambers.

Cumulated Index Medicus. Chicago: American Medical Association. (Formerly *Quarterly Cumulative Index Medicus;* contains a comprehensive list of abbreviation of journals and other publications.)

Current Abbreviations (Shankle). New York: H. V. Wilson.

Current List of Medical Literature. Washington. D.C.: National Library of Medicine. (Contains a comprehensive list of medical abbreviations.)

Current Medical Information and Terminology. Chicago: American Medical Association.

Current Procedural Terminology. Chicago: American Medical Association.

Directory of Medical Specialists (Marquis). Chicago: Who's Who. (Contains abbreviations of boards, certificates, medical schools, national and sectional societies.)

Discursive Dictionary of Health Care, A. Washington, D.C.: US Government Printing Office.

Dispensatory of the United States of America, The. (Contains an extensive list of abbreviations of publications.)

Doctors' Shorthand. Philadelphia: W. B. Saunders.

Everyman's Encyclopaedia. London: J. M. Dent.

Handbook of Chemistry and Physics. Cleveland, Ohio: Chemical Rubber Publishing.

International System (SI) Units, The, BS 3763. London: British Standards Institution.

Letters, Symbols, Signs and Abbreviations, BS 1991 part I General. London: British Standards Institution.

Medical Abbreviations: A Cross Reference Dictionary. Ann Arbor, Mich.: Michigan Occupational Therapy Association.

Medical Directory, The. London: Churchill.

Medical Physics, vol. II. Chicago: Year Book Publishers.

Medical Spelling Guide (Johnson). Springfield, Ill.: Charles C. Thomas.

Medical Terminology Made Easy (JeHarned). Berwyn, Ill.: Physicians Record Co.

Medical Word Book, The — A Spelling and Vocabulary Guide to Medical Transcription (Sloane). Philadelphia: W. B. Saunders.

Merck Index. Rahway, N.J.: Merck.

Scientific and Technical Definitions (Zimmerman and Levine). Industrial Research Service.

Stylebook]Editorial Manual: Chicago: American Medical Association.

Understanding Medical Terminology (Clare). St Louis, Mo: Catholic Hospital Association.

Units, Symbols and Abbreviations: A Guide for Biological and Medical Editors and Authors: London: Royal Society of Medicine.

Webster's Medical Speller. Springfield, Mass.: G. & C. Merriam.

Webster's New International Dictionary. Springfield, Mass.: G. & C. Merriam.

Whitaker's Almanack. London: J. Whitaker.

Who's Who. London: A. & C. Black.

World List of Scientific Periodicals. London: Butterworths.

World Medical Periodicals. London: British Medical Association.